LEUKAEMIA UNVEILED

Dedicated to you, Daddy

LEUKAEMIA UNVEILED

A teenager's battle with a formidable disease

CHANEL WEWEGE

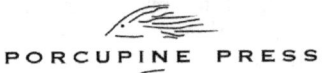

PORCUPINE PRESS

Johannesburg, South Africa

Copyright © Chanel Wewege 2013

ISBN-13: 978-1518646713 | ISBN-10: 1518646719

Published by Porcupine Press
PO Box 2756
Pinegowrie, 2123
South Africa
info@porcupinepress.co.za
www.porcupinepress.co.za

Cover designed by Wim Rheeder: wim@wimrheeder.co.za
Set in 10.5 point on 14.5 point, Minion Pro
Printed by CreateSpace

Contents

Author's Note

THIS is a true story of a battle I have won against a disease called: AML, Acute Myeloid Leukemia. It's a tale of faith, love and hope to you, the reader of this book. Whatever challenges you may be facing, may they be made small by your courage. I hope that this book will help you *face your fears* and know that this journey was chosen for you. You may not realise it now, but you will. God will *never* give you a challenge that you cannot handle. He knows you and your abilities. Always remember that.

In these pages you will learn of my experience with Cancer and how I dealt with it. You will find many testimonials about wonderful people I encountered along the way. I hope you enjoy this book and that it helps you.

Sincerely yours,

Chanel Wewege

Glossary of Medical Terms

From the National Bone Marrow Transplant Link

ADJUVANT chemotherapy—Drugs used to kill cancer cells. They are given with other treatments, such as surgery or radiation, to destroy areas of tumour.

Allogeneic transplant—The person donating the bone marrow or stem cells is a closely matched family member, usually a brother or sister. Or the person donating the bone marrow is a closely matched unrelated donor.

Alopecia—A partial or complete hair loss, usually a temporary side effect of the chemotherapy.

Anemia—A condition that occurs when the body's red blood cell count is low.

Antibody—A protein produced by the white blood cells (leukocytes) to battle foreign substances that enter the body, such as bacteria.

Antigen—A foreign substance that induces the production of antibodies.

Apheresis—The peripheral blood stem cell collection process in which blood is taken from a patient and circulated through a machine that separates out stem cells. The remaining cells are returned to the patient.

Appeal—Application for review of records, medical history, insurance claim.

Autologous transplant—The patient donates his/her own bone marrow or stem cells prior to treatment for reinfusion later after high doses of chemotherapy and/or radiation.

Bone marrow—The spongy tissue found in the cavities of the body's bones where all blood cells are produced.

Bone marrow harvest—The procedure of collecting stem cells from the bone marrow.

Bone marrow transplant (BMT)—A procedure developed to treat some forms of cancer and other diseases. There are several types of BMT's, depending on who donates the marrow (see Autologous, Allogeneic, and Syngeneic). Stem cells are removed from the bone marrow for transplant.

Cancer cells—Uncontrolled growth of abnormal cells in the body. Cancer cells can grow, divide, and invade normal tissue in the body.

Cell—The basic building block of life. In your blood, you will find many different types of these.

Central line or central venous catheter—A small, plastic tube inserted in a large vein to inject or remove fluids. The central line used in stem cell transplant allows blood samples to be drawn, drugs to be given, and the actual transplant to occur with little discomfort.

Chemotherapy—Treatment with one or more anticancer drugs to try to stop or slow the growth of cancer cells.

Clinical trials—Long-term research studies that test cancer treatment.

Colony stimulating factor—The drug given to autologous stem cell transplant patients before and during the harvest to increase the number of stem cells in the blood. It is also given to allogeneic donors to increase the number of cells in the circulating blood so they can be collected for transplant. Also called growth factor.

Complete Blood Count (CBC)—A blood test done in a laboratory to find out the number of red blood cells (RBC's), white blood cells (WBC's), platelets, hemoglobin, and hematocrit in your blood. These blood cells are made in the marrow of your bones.

Conditioning—A phase in the bone marrow/stem cell transplant process designed to destroy cancer cells more chemotherapy. Conditioning involves combining high doses of chemotherapy and/ or radiation.

Cord blood—Blood found in the umbilical cord.

Cord blood transplant—A procedure where umbilical blood stem cells are used in a stem cell transplant.

CT (Confirmatory Typing)—This test confirms the HLA compatibility of the donor and the patient and is performed on all potential family or unrelated donors. DNA—One of the nucleic acids found in the nucleus of the cell. It contains the information that allows a cell to grow and divide and become a unique (or particular type of) cell.

Engraftment—Process in which transplanted stem cells begin to grow in the recipient's bone marrow and produce new white blood cells, red blood cells, and platelets.

Erythrocytes—Red blood cells that carry oxygen.

Genes—Found in the nucleus of the cell. They contain the hereditary information that is passed on from cell to cell. Graft failure—Complication after a transplant in which the stem cells do not grow in the recipient's bone marrow and do not produce new white blood cells, red blood cells, and platelets.

Graft-versus-host disease (GVHD)—A condition where transplanted stem cells may react against the patient's body. Symptoms may range from a minor skin rash to more serious problems resulting in lifethreatening conditions.

Growth factor—(see Colony stimulating factor)

Harvest—(see Stem cell retrieval)

Hematocrit—The proportion of the blood that consists of packed red blood cells.

Hematologist—A doctor who specializes in the diseases of the blood.

Hematopoietic stem cells—Cells that mature into one of three types of blood cells: white blood cells, red blood cells, or platelets.

Hemoglobin—The part of the red blood cell which carries oxygen.

HLA (Human Leukocyte Antigen)— Antigens found on a person's cells that help the body to identify its own cells from invading or foreign cells.

HLA typing—The identification of a person's key antigens used for identifying compatible donors.

Immune compromised—A condition in which the patient has a much higher risk of infection due to a weak immune system.

Immune system—The group of organs and cells in the body that fight infection and other diseases.

Immunosuppressed—Lowered resistance to disease. It may be a temporary condition caused by a lowered white blood cell count or a side effect of receiving chemotherapy.

Informed consent—Hospital form, signed by the patient, which documents an understanding of medical procedures.

Infusion—Slow introduction of fluid into a vein referred to as an IV (intravenous).

Intravenous—Within a vein; into the vein.

Leukocytes—White blood cells that fight infection.

Lymphocytes—A type of white blood cell that is part of the immune system.

Metastasis—The spread of cancer from one part of the body to another.

Mobilization—Moving more stem cells from the bone marrow into the blood stream through chemotherapy and/or a growth factor.

MUD—Matched unrelated donor.

Oncologist—A doctor who specializes in the study and treatment of cancer.

Patient advocate—A person who acts in the best interest of the patient or serves the patient's needs and may act on his/her behalf.

Peripheral Blood Stem Cells (PBSC)— Stem cells that circulate in the blood.

Peripheral Blood Stem Cell Transplant— Stem cells are removed from the blood and infused after high-dose chemotherapy. This can be done for both autologous and allogeneic transplants.

Platelets—Blood cells that act as clotting agents to prevent bleeding.

Prognosis—The predicted or likely outcome.

Protocol—A specifically designed treatment plan.

Purging—The process of removing certain types of cells from the stem cell product before transplanting it to a patient. In autologous transplants, marrow may be purged of lingering cancer cells.

Radiation—Treatment to kill cancer cells using high-energy rays from x-rays, electron beams, or radioactive isotopes.

Red blood cells (RBC)—Cells carrying oxygen to all parts of the body (erythrocytes).

Reimbursement—Refund, being paid back for monies used out of pocket.

Reinfusion—The return of healthy stem cells into the transplant recipient's body.

Relapse—The return of cancer after a period of being cancer-free.

Remission—Complete or partial disappearance of cancer cells and symptoms.

Rescue process—Another term for a stem cell transplant. The re-infusion of healthy stem cells following high doses of chemotherapy or radiation.

Staging—The process of determining and describing the extent of the cancer.

Stem cell—The "parent cell." Every type of blood cell in the body begins its life as a stem cell. The stem cells then divide and form the different cells that make up the blood and immune system. Stem cells are found in both the bone marrow and circulating blood.

Stem cell retrieval—The process of collecting stem cells from the circulating blood stream following administration of growth factors to increase their numbers. (Also called harvest).

Stem cell transplant—(see Peripheral blood stem cell transplant).

Syngeneic transplant—The person donating the bone marrow or stem cells is an identical twin.

Thrombocytopenia—Low platelet count.

Transfusion—The transferring of blood or blood products directly into a vein or artery.

White blood cells (WBC)—Cells that help fight infection and disease (leukocytes).

Prologue

A S I lie in this prison-like room, in this cold bed, I am filled with fear as well as hope. The pre-med has calmed the chaos in my mind. I look up curiously as they assemble the drip that will, in a matter of hours either save my life or kill me. I cannot say that I remember everything but I do remember as though it were just yesterday that my life as a normal teenager was put on hold. Today, I will have an allogeneic transplant. This is also known as a bone-marrow transplant but with a perfect match. I am lucky and grateful to be able to have this choice. My journey will teach me so many vital lessons that I will use in my life. This illness will bring me closer to my family and teach me to never take anything for granted, *ever again*. You will live through these days with me in every page of this book. I am about to take you to a dark place that will forever remain a part of me, a time when I had to fight like I had never fought before…

This is my story.

Dr. Nel has a typical girl next door look, with dark brown hair which she wears in a bob. It is somewhat untidy but in a cute, sophisticated way. It gives you the impression that she's been running her fingers through it while trying to figure something out. Her skin is fair and she has a natural blush on the apple of both cheeks. Her lips are stained a subtle scarlet and her eyes seem to rest gently on your soul. She is feminine and graceful and is wearing a skirt and printed blouse, covered by a white coat that acts like an overall identifying her status. Her voice is very soft and her body language exudes empathy. Her degree is in haematology and oncology. In this case she is an assistant doctor to the head of the haematology department at Groote Schuur Hospital, Dr. Neil Littleton.

He's a good looking gentleman, with dusty blonde hair. A typical movie star doctor, if you know what I mean. He exudes confidence as he walks along the passages of the hospital. My first impression of him is pleasantly memorable. I immediately feel safe in his capable presence. What strikes me most is his sense of humour. He has the ability to make you laugh at a life-threatening illness. This is one of the key elements that will get me through the darker days.

Dr. Nel is assigned to monitor my progress during the transplant. Concentrating intensely on the task at hand, she sits in the grey chair not far from my bed staring at the drip, then back at me, then back at her clipboard again. I vaguely see her jotting something down. The pre-meds have impaired my senses. I can only imagine this whole thing from her perspective, how it must feel to have the responsibility of someone else's life in your hands, *knowing* that this drip may turn into a lethal injection rather than an antidote to the poisonous Cancer that has consumed my body. She proceeds as she was trained to do. All of those years in medical school have brought her to this point today, to this specific patient in this crucial moment. I am not her only patient and I will not be her last, yet I am her number one priority right now.

My attention turns to the bag attached to the drip stand as we share the moment of watching the first drop of liquid separate itself from the bag and drip into the pipe way. My eyes enthusiastically follow after it as it runs through the tube toward my vein, eventually making its way into my body. At this point I am afraid, despite what I have been through this year, I am not sure I have been this scared before. I look around the room, my movement causes dizziness but I force myself to stay conscious. My fingers grip the white blanket and I feel its texture. It is rough, yet comforting. I lift my hand to touch my head, it's the second time my hair has fallen out due to chemotherapy. I run my fingers down my face. I can feel the bones of my eye sockets. I quickly pull my hand away and back down next to me. There are machines everywhere. My body is extremely weak and my immune system barely exists anymore. Dr Nel continues to monitor my every move. I can't help but feel like a science project; I am sedated and calm, yet agitated, confused and hopeful all at the same time. This surreal state of mind is terrifying. It just doesn't feel real, more like a nightmare, I blink and realise how real it really is, very real. I could die.

I try to lift my hand again but this time it falls back down onto the sheets by itself with a light thump beside me. I look at my hand thinking, *so this is what it feels like to be completely helpless and emotionally paralysed.*

During the course of this year I have come to know too well what this emotional paralysis feels like. Even if this procedure is successful, I know that it does not end here. Today, I weigh in at roughly 35 kg. It hurts just to lie down in this bed because it feels as though there is nothing separating my skin from my bones anymore. My breathing is irregular, yet my heart beat is constant. I hear the heart monitor. Beep, beep, beep…

Chapter 1

How it all began

IT was in December 2004 when my life changed so suddenly. I am a healthy young lady with a lot of ambition and I'm a bit of a dreamer. We are a family of five; my mom, my dad, two brothers Sheldon (age 15), Daine (age 9) and myself (age 17). We're not rich but we love each other and that's all that matters. My report card shows my advancement to Grade 11. Excitement has filled my heart and the tremendous feeling of moving forward lightly caresses my soul.

A few weeks prior to school and year end I start experiencing flu-like symptoms; headaches and feeling weak and it doesn't improve. It's as if it's become normal to wake up tired and despondent these days. Along with this constant lethargic feeling, I have now developed a blister on the back of my ankle caused by the leather of my school shoe and it just won't heal. Irritated by the pain and desperate to feel well again, I ask mom to make an appointment for me to see our family G.P. He examines me and says that I am indeed coming down with the flu and that my immune system is run down. This may be the reason the wound is taking so long to heal. He prescribes a course of antibiotics as well as a container of pain tablets and antibacterial ointment to put onto the wound.

'Finish the five-day course and take the pain pills when necessary.' He says, reassuring me that I will be back to normal in no time. Relieved and trusting I left his office, already feeling better. As advised, I finish the antibiotic course and started to feel human again.

There was still the entire holiday to get through as well as the New Year's party my friends and I had been planning to attend for months. Mom helps with the arrangements for me to go up to Pretoria to visit her family for the first half of the holidays. I am looking forward to getting away, seeing new people and being in a different environment. A couple of days later, mom and dad drive me to the Greyhound bus station so I can commence my trip to Pretoria. I assure my parents that I will keep in contact with them throughout my trip and see them soon. Off to Pretoria I go.

The days there are filled with fun and laughter except for one particular day, the day that would be the beginning of my terrible journey. My aunt's family and I decide to go grocery shopping. We have both trolleys almost full when all of the sudden I feel this really strange tingle rush through my body and I am paralysed. It's almost as though someone has poured cement over my body and it has dried before I have time to get away. Frozen in time, I can feel myself slowly collapse to the floor. It becomes completely impossible for me to control my body at this point.

I remember knowing and feeling exactly what was happening to me but being completely immobilised and not able to stop it.

I fall into some display boxes in the corner of one of the isles and then onto the floor. Everything around me is spinning and all I can hear are echoes while people frantically try to lift me up from the ground. My eyes are open and I can see them, but I am completely numb. All of this happens within a few seconds and Aunty Tracy desperately helps me back up onto my feet.

''Are you alright?' she asks frantically, completely shocked by what had just happened.

I try to stand up straight, disorientated and confused. Aunty Tracy rushes me to the nearest pharmacy. The chemist listens to the story and suspects that my blood pressure is low. She then proceeds to take a blood pressure test. It does appear to be just a little low, but according to her, I have nothing to worry about. So, after buying a cold drink for sugar we go on our merry way not too concerned about the incident. Back at the house I go up to the room to lie down after calling my parents regarding the days' events. That night I develop an excruciating pain on the back side of my hip and it moves its way to my lower back and eventually it becomes hard for me to breathe normally. My body just starts feeling strange again. By this point I am anxious and scared. Aunty Tracy walks in to check on me, and I tell her about this new symptom. She gives me her phone to call my parents again. After talking to them I feel so much better and I wipe away my tears, missing my family terribly and happy to be going home in the morning.

I take something for the pain and before falling asleep I say a silent prayer to God asking for this pain to go away and that I am afraid it is something serious. Natural instinct is an amazing human ability instilled in all of us. It is a gift, because despite what the chemist had told us and the fact that the pain medication is helping somewhat, I can still feel that something is very wrong with me. It is time for me to go back home to Port Elizabeth. I have missed my mom, dad and brothers greatly and have many stories to tell them about my trip. So, I say my goodbyes and off I go back to the bus station.

The trip back home is unpleasant as the pain in my lower back is still there and worsening. Seeing mom, dad and the boys again makes me smile and I run into their arms. While we walk to the car I tell them all about the pain and what had happened to me on that horrid day in the shop. When we get home, I go to my room and throw my bags onto the floor as I am far too tired to unpack. I wash my hands, and walk into the kitchen to see what mom is making for dinner. It feels so good to be home and to enjoy a meal with my family again.

Now that I'm back home, I need to put all negative thoughts behind me. St Francis Bay is waiting and New Year is going to be awesome. I wasn't going to let this spoil my fun. Finally, the day arrives and I'm ready and packed for the New Year's trip to St Francis Bay.

I will not think about or even mention what happened on that dreadful day in the shop.

I'll be meeting up with my cousins and friends. It's a beautiful drive and soon we can see the green golf course that's right opposite the house that we're going to be staying in. We pull up into the driveway where our friends are standing around waiting. The girls and I hastily get out of the car. As soon as we say our goodbyes and our parents are gone we go and get settled in. We spend our days exploring the town, having fun on the beach, braais, parties and talking all night. We are all looking forward to the big New Year's Eve party featuring my favorite bands: Evanescence and Seether.

The day before the big event we all decide to go down to the beach. We settle down at a pleasing spot on the sand and I watch as the water races up onto the beach and then back again into the deep, turquoise sea. Starting to feel unusually tired and weak, I lie down and place a towel over my face to block out the sharp rays of the sun. It honestly feels as though my energy is unwillingly being drained from me through some type of invisible device.

Such a strange feeling I think.

I must have dozed off for a second and I hear echoing voices. I sit up and there's a sharp pain that runs through my head. I'm not feeling great and tell the girls that I'd like to go back to the house.

Looking back now, I must have been so irritating to be around.

I can barely remember walking back to the house from the beach. As soon as my head hits the pillow I fall asleep. I open my eyes only to find it's late afternoon and I have an incredibly dry mouth and am craving water. As I sit up, I begin to feel a bit dizzy and nauseous.

How long have I been sleeping?

I hear voices on the deck and so I peep out of the window and see my friends chilling outside, watching the beautiful orange sky. The sun is already starting to set. I walk out of the room and into the bathroom. Catching a glimpse of myself in the mirror, I notice how pale I am. I splash some cold water from the tap onto my face and look into the mirror again. I take a sip of water. 'What's up with you babe?' shouts Chavonne from across the deck while in mid-conversation with one of the girls.

'That's the thing, I don't know. No matter how long I had been asleep for, I still feel as though I could go right back to bed and sleep forever.'

The fire is on the go and we are going to braai some meat for dinner. I can't say I have much of an appetite and I have unintentionally been skipping a lot of meals lately.

It is the big night and on the way there, butterflies set in and I can barely speak I am so excited. Tonight I will see *Evanescence* live for the first time. My idol and my muse. With so many people around, I soon get lost in the crowd and I'm alone. I'm not too fazed by this and I decide to approach the stage to get a closer look.

Ouch!

This pain is beginning to nag at me again. I look up as Amy Lee walks onto the stage and my heart soars. This is one of the most amazing moments of my life. I find a place in the corner and just stand there for a while, watching her perform. It is enchanting.

Seether takes the stage as well and they sing '*Broken*' together. It's so beautiful. I suddenly feel warm liquid run down my legs. Frightened and confused I stand dead still and look down but because I am wearing a pair of black pants, I cannot see anything. It just keeps pouring out of me and I can barely move. Frightened, I look around to see where the nearest toilet facility is. I see a row of green mobile toilets not too far from where I'm standing and I rush toward them as fast as I can. I'm in luck as one of them is available.

It's so dark inside the cubicle I can't see my own hand in front of my face. I soon realise that there isn't any toilet paper. Annoyed and feeling disgusted I walk out and stand for a while trying to find my bearings. Just then, the girls walk by laughing and chatting. I try to call out to them to help me but they just shout something back to me that I can't make out and carry on walking and laughing. I make a decision there and then to find a way back to the house. I need to try and figure out what's going on. As I touch my inner thigh and then lift my hand back up, I look down and see that my fingers are covered in bright red blood. I now realise that the warm liquid running down my legs is blood.

The first thing I think is that I must have my period again this month. It's impossible, I have just finished a week ago. I stand there, distressed and confused. I have to try and get someone's attention to help me get back to the house. I walk around searching for someone I know. I am so scared.

Relieved, I see my dad's cousin Luke across the field. I walk up to him and immediately start to tell him what is happening and that I need to get back to the house and he offers to take me. On the way, I remember that we ran out of toilet paper at the house and all the shops are closed. We drive past a house and see people having a house party. We stop to ask if I can use their bathroom. At this point, I am very weak. All I want is to clean myself and sleep. We knock on the door and they are so friendly. They lead me to the bathroom and I rush in. I can actually feel the blood pouring out of me. It is a different type of blood to a normal period.

This blood is bright red; it's new, clean blood. I grab as much toilet paper as I can and try to stop the bleeding. I wash my hands and then take a toilet roll from the basket next to the toilet and put it into my handbag. I feel bad for just taking it but I have no choice. We say thank you and leave.

We arrive at the house and all I want to do is shower and sleep. As I walk towards the front door, I see that some people are standing around with my friends at a fire. Luke makes sure I am safe and sound before he leaves. I immediately jump into the shower. Blood flows down the drain along with the warm water. I start to cry and pray. I ask why this is happening to me, I'm so afraid. I change into my pajamas, take as much toilet paper as I can and place it between my legs to block the blood flow, then I curl up into a little ball on the bed and fall asleep.

I am woken up by loud voices and the noise of the girls coming back from the party. Once again, I don't know for how long I have been asleep. My head feels enormous and it's throbbing. I turn onto my other side and I see a huge puddle of blood on the sheets. I have bled right through the large wad of toilet paper. The girls are shocked and all come to help me. I can barely get up, I am so weak. I wipe the blood with a towel and lie one of my t-shirts over the stained area. After going to the bathroom and placing fresh toilet paper between my legs, I fall back onto the bed and go back to sleep.

The next morning I wake up with a terrible headache and an earache too. I cannot cope with this. I feel dirty and immediately go and take a shower. I soak the drenched sheet and t-shirt in some soap in the basin while I get dressed, then go back to wash it properly and hang it up outside. Luckily, the bleeding had subsided to a normal period flow and I am now able to control it using normal sanitary ware, thanks to one of the girls' toiletry bags. After my shower and a change of clothes, I'm starting to feel myself again. I have no idea of how long I've been asleep. I walk slowly down stairs and everyone greets me. It's almost afternoon. The girls are dressed and ready for the beach. I wonder how I slept through the noise. This afternoon our parents will come to fetch us. Nobody else wants to go home yet, except for me. I can't wait to be at home, to sleep in my own bed again.

The drive home seems so long, I say nothing as everyone

else babbles on. I open the door to my bedroom and just fall onto my bed.

The next morning I wake up with the same pounding headache. I decide to get up and drink a glass of water. My mind is telling me to stand up but my body has other ideas. I just don't feel right and I am also experiencing dizziness. I walk to the bathroom to take a bath. I hear mom in the kitchen, making breakfast. My brothers are probably still asleep. I wonder where dad is. I walk out of my room and into the bathroom, closing the bathroom door behind me. I turn on the taps and while taking my clothes off, I notice a large bruise on my thigh; must have been from St Francis. I take my top off slowly as I am still rather dizzy and see another huge bruise on my upper arm, near my bicep. This is starting to feel strange. I turn off the taps and check the temperature of the water with my fingertips before climbing into the bath. I sit down.

It hurts a bit to just sit in the bath, almost as though my bottom is also bruised.

I take the soap and start to wash my body. Things seem to be happening in slow motion and my reactions seem somewhat impaired.

What is going on with me?

I finish my bath and pull out the plug. I stand up slowly and reach for the towel, almost falling over. I quickly grab the rail and attempt to stand up straight again. Weird... I wrap the towel around my body and step out of the bath cautiously. I open the door and walk to my bedroom to get dressed.

'Mom, would you please come and look at this?' I call out.

Mom comes walking in looking concerned. I take off my towel and show her my new bruises; she notices another big one at the back of my leg behind my knee.

'That's not right,' she says.

I did tell her about the dizziness and how I almost fell when I stood up to get out of the bath.

'I think I need to see another doctor, Mom.' I say softly. 'Yes, I agree.' She replies. 'We will book an appointment for you next week.'

Chapter 2

The realisation

It is about three days later and mom asks from the kitchen, 'How's your earache?'

'It's okay,' I shout back. 'But now I have that pain in my back again.' An irritating, nagging ache in my lower hip area.

As we are chatting we hear the front gate open. It is Uncle Marco, mom's brother, and behind him is his wife, my Aunty Charmaine and Shirley, my grandmother on my mother's side.

'Shirls is here!' I shout.

Shirley was a very big part of my life as I was growing up. I looked up to her and loved her with all my heart. She was like a second mother to me.

They walk into the house and Uncle Marco asks where mom and dad are. It isn't the usual friendly hello that I am used to and concern sets in. We are a very close family and we make it known that we are always happy to see each other. Shirley is holding a large brown envelope.

What is this all about?

Mom comes walking in from the kitchen smiling and greeting everyone just as dad walks out from their bedroom.

Shirley asks mom to follow her to the room as she has something to tell her. She goes in the direction of the bedroom, still holding the envelope. Mom follows her, concerned and naturally inquisitive. Uncle Marco gives dad a brief explanation of what is really going on.

'We've just come from the doctor,' says Uncle Marco. 'Those are Shirls' X-rays in the brown envelope.'

He could barely finish his sentence when we hear mom screaming from the room.

'NO! No, please, I can't lose you!'

Mom comes running from the passage into Uncle Marco's arms. We are all so shocked and confused. Then Shirley breaks the news to us slowly. She has been diagnosed with liver and lung cancer. There is nothing more that the doctors can do for her. It is at a very advanced stage and not even chemotherapy can help. I think mom is going to faint. Dad holds her so tight. Shirley is such a strong woman. I didn't cry that day. I love Shirls with all my heart, she helped raise me but I can't cry, the tears refuse to flow. I give her a huge hug and breathe her in. I guess I don't fully understand the magnitude of the news. Mom suggests that Shirley should stay with us so that we can at least look after her and make her as happy as possible here close with her family. I love this idea.

Aunty Charmaine and Uncle Marco walk Shirley to their car. As we all walk out with her, it starts to drizzle. She turns to mom and with a beautiful smile starts singing 'Rain drops are falling on my head.' Mom bursts into tears and holds her tightly. We have so many questions.

The next day Shirls arrives with her stuff and mom sets her

up in the main bedroom. She is her normal self, bubbly and independent but she seems tired and weak. She tells mom she'd like to lie down for a while. All I want is to be close to her, so I go and lie next to her on the bed. I don't say a single word. I guess I don't really know how to act. I spend my nights next to her in this way. There is medication that she needs to take and her body is getting weaker and weaker by the day. Mom makes her glucose liquid to drink and forces her to eat. She sleeps a lot and I stay with her as long as I can while she is awake.

Shirley is becoming disorientated and different. It kills mom to see her this way. On the last night I see her, she gives me two rings from her fingers. She has lost so much weight that it is hard to believe she was once a very well groomed and beautiful lady. She was very eccentric and never dull. On one hand she only wore gold: a gold watch, three gold rings and one single gold band. On the other hand she just wore silver: five silver bangles, two silver rings and one single silver band. She gave me the two single bands; one silver and the other gold.

I still wear them today and I have never taken them off.

She also gives me her legendary silver bangles. You would know Shirley was around by the faint whispering melodies and the tingling of her bangles. She always smelled of a sweet floral fragrance. Her shoes matched her outfits and her hair and make-up were always done. This was the Shirley I was going to miss forever, the one who would give me advice about boys and always back me up in front of my parents.

When Shirley was still well, I would spend weekends at her place. We would watch All My Children and Generations together and talk about anything and everything. She always told me that I was special, that I was different and would amount to something very great one day. She would make me feel so shy, claiming that I was the most beautiful girl in the world. At that age I believed her *just* because she was 'Shirley'.

She hands me the jewelry and tells me to always keep it safe. I give her a kiss on her cheek and cuddle up next to her and fall asleep. Suddenly, I wake up with this excruciating pain in my lower back. I try to crawl out of bed. Shirley is lying next to me and the house is silent. I scream out in agony and try to get up to wake my parents. I am drooling from the pain and biting my lip. My breathing starts to alter and I can feel the pain running up my spine. Nothing eases it, not sitting, standing, or lying down. It's getting worse.

'Mom! It hurts! Please! I can't wait till next week to see the doctor. I promise you. I can't take this pain! Please! Help me.'

At this point I am crawling on the ground and mom and dad are trying to help me to my feet. Sheldon is still in bed and is told to stay home with Shirls while mom, dad, Daine and I get into the car and drive to the hospital.

Rushing into the Emergency Trauma Ward at Greenacres Hospital Port Elizabeth, a million thoughts are running through my mind and I'm confused and scared. I am in so much pain I crunch down to hold my cries in while we wait for someone to assist us. I don't understand why my hip is paining so much. It is excruciating, it hurts really badly. The hospital smells of disinfectant and we are surrounded by sick and hurt people who need medical assistance. The nurse calls my surname: *Miss Wewege*. Mom helps me up from the chair. It's so hard to walk and just concentrating on putting one foot in front of the other is almost impossible. The nurses take me to an examination bed behind a white curtain. They close it slightly. Florescent lights, the sound of beeping heart monitors and doctors talking to patients fill my ears. The nurse takes my temperature and blood pressure while we wait for the doctor to arrive.

'We suspect it might be a muscle spasm' says the nurse. 'Have you been doing any physically challenging activities this holiday?' she continues. 'Well, I did go to Gold Reef City while I was up in Johannesburg if that counts' I said breathlessly, 'I went on many rides.'

Mom informs the nurse about the fainting incident. I am then injected with Voltaren which eases the pain almost immediately. Already starting to feel better, the consensus is that I go home to rest and if the pain increases, I am to come back later in the day for more tests. Agreeing with the sisters, my parents, Daine and I prepare to leave. Just as I'm about to be sent home with some Myprodol for the pain I guess, when a blonde lady walks by the doorway glancing quickly into the room and at me. She stops steps back and walks into the room.

She immediately introduces herself as Dr. Swart. She reaches for my hand, places her index finger on my wrist and begins counting silently. She turns to mom and asks whether I am usually this pale. Mom looks over at me and back at the doctor and tells her that I am not usually so pale or tired. Dr. Swart then takes a blood sugar test, warns me briefly of the prick and then takes the blood sample with her.

'Go home and rest,' she says in a gentle tone. 'We will call you with the results as soon as we have them.'

We wonder about her lack of explanation but too tired to ask for one, we eventually leave to go home. I walk into the house and collapse on the couch and fall asleep. Thirty minutes or so later, I am woken by the sound of the cell phone ringing.

'Yes, okay. Is it serious doctor?' Mom asks. 'Okay.'

She walks over to the couch, to wake me.

'Come on girl.' she says. 'We have to pack some clothes for

you because you will be staying over in the hospital for a while.'

I remember being frightened by the tone in her voice and perhaps the fact that she spoke with tears in her eyes. Dad quickly grabs his car keys, mom takes my bag of clothes and we are on our way back to the hospital. The drive seems to take forever. Everyone is quiet, nobody says a word. The sun has started to rise and there is a sharp glare in my eyes. I like it. Daine sits next to me also staring out the window. His timid little body perched next to mine. I wonder what must be going through his mind and at nine years old, if he even understands. Then I turn to my parents and wonder if they understand. Finally I look to myself, linking my fingers together and realising that not even I understand.

We get to the hospital and walk through the glass doors to the reception. Mom nervously tells the receptionist about the call she had received. She gets up and leads us into a tiny office.

'Dr. Wickens will be with you shortly.' She assures us.

Normal human behaviour forces us to look around the room scoping and twiddle our thumbs waiting in anticipation for the reason of why we have been summoned back to the hospital. Just

Dr. Wickens enters the room and closes the door firmly behind him.

'Mr. and Mrs. Wewege, I am not going to beat around the bush.' he says. Turning towards me he continues, 'Your daughter is very sick.'

Frightened and shocked, I turn to look at mom and dad. I can see my mom's face filled with worry, pain and fear. Without thinking, I get up and walk out of the room. Daine follows me.

I find my way to a cubicle and sit down on the chair. Daine sits closely next to me. He too is scared. His little hand finds mine and we wait there together. All of a sudden I hear my mom scream, '*NO!*'

I hear her crying and the commotion in the room behind that brown door is loud. Daine stands up and starts pacing. The fear in his eyes echoed in mine. 'Why is mom screaming Nelly?' he asks me, beginning to cry. It must have taken no longer than five minutes before the door flew open and my parents come walking towards us. That moment felt like hours. I didn't know how to answer Daine. It was me they were talking about. I was very sick, I was the one mom was screaming for, *me*. I fell silent and just waited. Everything went back to real time and mom is running towards me. Dad has tears in his eyes and comes to sit next to me and holds my hand.

'Everything will be okay. People survive this illness all the time' says mom.

I think she's trying to re-assure herself more than me. I still have no idea what is happening and time starts to drag again. Finally, the nurse comes in to explain my medical diagnosis to *me*. 'Chanel, you have AML, Acute Myeloid Leukemia' she says. Daine turns to me and asks in a sad, concerned tone; 'Are you going to die Nelly?'

I look to the nurse for an answer as I myself become overwhelmed with a feeling of deep sadness. It truly felt as though time stood still just for me. Everyone else was moving and talking and all I could hear was white noise and vague vibrations. The nurse takes my hand: 'Leukemia is a curable illness and we will be doing all that we can to save your life.'

Leukemia is Cancer I think to myself. I feel my body go tingly and numb. Dr. Wickens has requested that I book into hospital immediately for treatment. Leukemia is cancer of the blood or bone marrow. Uncontrolled growth of abnormal cells in the body, cancer cells can grow, divide, and invade normal tissue in the body. In this type of illness, there is no time to waste and each minute another healthy cell dies in my body.

I ask if we can go outside for a while until the hospital admission arrangements are taken care of. Permission is granted. We are different to who we were thirty minutes ago. We take a walk outside in the fresh morning air. The sun is bright and magnificent as it peers through the clouds to greet me, touching my face like a warm hand, almost saying that everything is going to be okay. So many questions are running through my mind and my parents are saying theirs out loud.

'It's going to be okay Johnny,' says mom. 'We just need to pray and be there for each other.' She says with complete acceptance of the journey to come. Dad agrees with her and walks up to me, grabbing me in his arms. Confused, afraid and unsure, we walk back into the hospital. Dad and mom start calling the family while the arrangements for my admittance to St. George's Hospital are made. I feel as though this is all just a bad dream and I'll wake up soon. I take a couple of deep breathes and blink a few times. This seems to help my brain accept that this is reality and I must prepare myself for what lies ahead.

A nurse wheels me into the room in which my journey with this illness shall begin. It's a small, cozy room with blue curtains. There's a prominent smell of disinfectant in the air. Above my bed are two name tags: C. Wewege, and the other Dr. Musson. Mom opens the curtains and the sun greets us again. Dr. Musson walks in to get acquainted with us and to try his best to make my diagnosis sound a little better than what it actually is. He is a soft-spoken man with gentle hands and a compassionate manner.

I can tell that he is both intelligent and knowledgeable in his explanation regarding the dark days to follow. I feel at ease. Mom and dad look at him with big eyes, studying his every move. Dr. Musson finishes talking to us and leaves the room.

There is a moment of silence and I cannot recall what he has said to us. I lie back on the pillow wondering when my family will arrive; my cousins, my aunts, everyone. I try not to focus on the fact that a nurse has just entered my room with a kidney dish, needles and an armband.

'We are going to set up a drip.' she says.

I hate needles. I know that this is going to hurt and that I am not familiar with all of these medical procedures. Mom and dad have just walked out of the room to get something to eat and drink. My appetite is the last thing on my mind as I am alone with her. She doesn't talk much, her hands do what she is trained to do and her expression remains the same. I ask her something silly like, 'Is it going to hurt?' She doesn't answer. I feel so utterly alone. She straps my arm tightly with the band and tells me to open and close my hand into a fist to stimulate the blood flow. She grips my right hand in her left one and taps the now prominent veins that are pulsing through my skin. She opens the needle packaging. It's a really thick needle with a pink rim and it's quite apparent how sharp it is as she pushes the hollow point into my vein. I am taken back by the rush of pain that runs up and down my arm. I gasp and she pulls the needle out and a white plastic tube is left behind in my vein. She breaks off a piece of surgical tape and sticks it across my hand, making sure the plastic needle is secure. She turns around for a second and I start to feel a warm sensation run down my fingertips. I look down and the blood is pouring out of the tiny hole she had just made. I scream. She immediately releases the band from my arm but at this point I am hysterical and she tries to calm me down.

Mom and dad come running into the room; my sheet is drenched in blood. She cleans up the mess, apologises and takes a number of alcohol swabs to clean the blood from my hand. A drip with a bag of saline is set up to flush my vein in preparation for the blood transfusion I must receive. She leaves the room unaware that those seconds will haunt me for the rest of my life. I cannot stand blood, bleeding and needles. Yet, it doesn't matter what I can and cannot stand because that was only the beginning. I hear familiar voices coming from far down the passage. Just then the same nurse returns holding a syringe, a closed needle and a tiny brown glass bottle. She opens and connects the needle to the syringe and then inserts the needlepoint into the tiny brown bottle without breaking the seal. She turns the bottle upside down and extracts a carefully measured amount of the liquid from the bottle into the syringe tube. It is clear that the precision of this task is important and that whatever this substance is, I am only allowed a little bit of it. She swabs my upper arm and injects the substance into my body. Ouch. It really stings and I immediately start to feel a rush of calmness run through my entire body which forces me to lie back onto the pillows.

'That was pethadene for the pain,' she says with a gentle smile. 'It will also help you to sleep.'

I am filled with a feeling of contentment and joy for some reason. I have never felt this way before and the pain in my lower back seems to have disappeared like a river that washes away a tin can. The voices grow louder and louder. Members of my family walk into the room. Abnormally happy, my first instinct is to greet them with a smile. I must seem like a complete neurotic weirdo to them at that moment. They all seem to arrive at the same time. Overwhelmed by their presence, I sit up and prepare to answer their questions. Aunty Jean, my dad's blonde sister with her soft skin and ever so scarlet lips, a hairdresser by profession and a loving, caring, strong woman is followed into the room by her husband. My Uncle Mark is a surfer, fitness fanatic and a respected estate agent in the city of Port Elizabeth. He also has a wonderful sense of humor. I see my cousins, their daughters, peep into my room, Chavonne, Shannon (my St Francis bay adventure accomplices) along with their two younger sisters Merle and Hannah. Merle is just like her dad, intelligent and business orientated. I swear that girl will grow up to be a doctor one day. Little Hannah, just a baby, is beautiful and fair like her mother with gorgeous big green eyes like her dad. I never looked at them as clearly as at this moment. Immediately everyone starts talking at the same time. It's like a flea market in this tiny room and a silly hint of embarrassment runs short lived through my mind. Then I realise that they are all here because they care and love me. Mom is crying on Aunty Jean's shoulder. Minutes later, my Uncle Marco, my mom's brother, his wife Charmaine, their daughter Leigh Ann and son Marco Jnr come into the room, devastated. The room is crowded and everyone is speaking at the same time.

'Where is Tim?' I ask. 'Has anyone told him?'

Tim was my boyfriend at the time. Shannon walks over to me, takes out her phone and types his name into her contact list. She brings the phone up to her ear and waits for an answer.

'Hello, Tim. Chanel just found out she has cancer. We are all here with her at St George's Hospital.'

He must have started laughing because she says it isn't a joke and that I have been diagnosed with leukemia. She ends the call. 'He is on his way' she says. Everyone has a turn to talk to me and there's a camera, photographs are being taken. My brother Sheldon is also here now. I am completely sedated and everything around me is a blur. My eyes are getting heavy and just as I want to fall asleep, Tim walks into the room. Everyone leaves and it is just Tim and I. He gives me a CD. It's Evanescence. I am ecstatic. He also hands me a portable CD player and earphones and we listen to track four together:

'*My Immortal*' by Evanescence

Songwriters: Amy Lee, Ben Moody, David Hodges

I'm so tired of being here, suppressed by all my childish fears
And if you have to leave, I wish that you would just leave
Your presence still lingers here and it won't leave me alone
These wounds won't seem to heal, this pain is just too real
There's just too much that time cannot erase

When you cried, I'd wipe away all of your tears
When you'd scream, I'd fight away all of your fears
And I held your hand through all of these years
But you still have all of me

You used to captivate me by your resonating light
Now, I'm bound by the life you left behind
Your face it haunts my once pleasant dreams
Your voice it chased away all the sanity in me

These wounds won't seem to heal, this pain is just too real
There's just too much that time cannot erase

When you cried, I'd wipe away all of your tears

When you'd scream, I'd fight away all of your fears
And I held your hand through all of these years
But you still have all of me

I've tried so hard to tell myself that you're gone
But though you're still with me, I've been alone all along

When you cried, I'd wipe away all of your tears
When you'd scream, I'd fight away all of your fears
And I held your hand through all of these years
But you still have all of me, me, me.

Three days later I am transferred to Tygerburg Hospital. As I get into the ambulance, the two medics give me a dolphin teddy signed with their names. I smile. They drive mom and me to the airport where we will be flown to Cape Town. The plane ride is terrible and I'm in so much pain. My ears hurt and I cannot hold in my cries. Mom holds me in her arms and tries to comfort me. "We get to Cape Town airport where another ambulance takes us to the hospital. We arrive at Tygerburg and I'm wheeled into the hospital. Dad and Tim have not arrived yet. They are driving up together.

A nurse shows us to my room. The wind howls through the corridors and I clutch mom's hand. My room is so cold and all that's on the bed is a white sheet. I immediately lie down, exhausted from the flight and still in terrible pain. My doctor is not available and I am going to have to spend the night without any prescribed pain medication. I feel my stomach muscles pull as the pain screams through my bones. I'm given another Panado but it doesn't work. Tim and dad arrive. The pain is getting worse and worse. This moment makes my parents realise the kind of agony I'm in. I sit up in my bed and grab my dad's body firmly, begging him to help me. Tears are pouring from my eyes as I scream in agony. There is nothing he can do, other than pray. I see tears in his eyes as he watches me helplessly. I start throwing up saliva every few minutes as the pain intensifies. I eventually crawl into a little ball and try and hum myself to sleep. Mom and dad have to find a place to rest. Tim stays and sleeps next to me on the floor. The nurses are also very concerned and they try everything they can to help me. *I can still feel that terrible pain if I really think back hard enough.*

The next day we are introduced to the doctor. He explains to us that this treatment can take anything from six months to a year. We are in for a long, hard battle. I am taken to have a bone-marrow biopsy. I start to cry, afraid of the unknown. Mom is taking it badly, I can see she just wants to break down but because she is so strong I can cope better. They give me a sedative and finally an injection for pain.

My body starts to become lame and I kind of can't lift my arms but at least the pain is subsiding. A lady comes to fetch me on a mobile bed. Mom, dad and Tim hold my hand as she rolls me away. I am frightened and ask her what is going to happen. I will be having my first bone-marrow biopsy she says. This is a test that will help them determine what doses of chemotherapy I will receive. As we roll toward the operating room I feel myself let go. The smell of this place is so strong and sterile. The doctor's instructions of how I should lie are vague to me. I turn to lie on my tummy with my arms tucked neatly beside me. I look up frightened and see the needle. I am told to relax.

How on earth am I supposed to relax with that needle? I feel a prick. 'Ouch!' But it's not that bad. The lady talks me through it. 'Chanel, that was the local anesthetic to numb the area that we are going to take the biopsy from.'

I am pricked a few times and I start to feel numb. I look up and am told to lie still. I feel the doctor's hand on my back and I know that she is inserting the bigger needle now. At first I do not feel a thing as the needle passes through the piece of skin numbed by the anesthetic. Then I start to feel the deepest and most excruciating pain as the needle pierces into my bone. I then feel this enormous pressure as the doctor pushes and twists the needle in and out of my bone. I scream out in agony and start to weep. My whole leg starts to pull stiffen as she pushes it in deeper and deeper. She eventually pulls it out for the last time, taking with her a tiny piece of my bone. She transfers it into a test tube and closes up the wound. I am left gasping and I have a massive headache. Relieved it is over, I attempt to sit up. The doctor shows me the piece of bone floating in a strange dense liquid. 'It looks like a worm.'

All I want to do now is sleep. I am wheeled back to my room. Exhausted and defeated I just want to be alone for a while. Dad and Tim come to say goodbye. I am sad but feel as though I have no more tears to cry. Mom and I are left behind. A dark feeling comes over me and I feel a sense of terrible loss. It hurts so much that I can feel myself fall apart. When I wake up mom and I are introduced to some of the nurses in the cancer ward. Mom asks if I would like to take a bath, I nod. After my bath it is night fall again. Sitting in the bed, mom starts to talk to me and I just stare at the wall. For days I ignore everyone as realisation sets in and I am forced to face my fears. Mom cries and I just lie there. She holds my hand but I don't respond.

' You are not being fair Chanel,' she says 'Don't do this, I am here with you. We are in this together my child. Snap out of it.'

Her voice sounds distant and I am dazed. I think I just need some time to adjust. There is a lot that I don't understand, a lot of unanswered questions. *I am in a cancer ward, I have cancer.* It's so difficult to come to terms with the fact that there's a huge chance I could die. I am told by the medical staff to prepare myself for a lot of pain. At just seventeen, how do I prepare myself for pain? I pray and pray each and every day, every moment that I can. I am closer to God than I have ever been.

The way I felt before, full of fear and anger is now gone and find myself feeling ready. Ready to face this disease and fight it with all that I have. It is as though something supernatural has come over me and I have snapped out of the hypnotic depressive state I was in. I turned to my mom and she didn't need to say a thing, she could see I was back.

Chapter 3

Days I Long to Forget

MOM lies next to me on a lazy boy chair every night. She falls asleep watching me and makes sure I am fine. The constant beep of the machines keeps me awake. I sit up in the silence and hear my mom's peaceful breathing. This is the only time she is content it seems, though I know her dreams have become nightmares and her thoughts have become consumed with this experience.

I close my eyes and I put myself in a better place, a place in the past. My mind is able to relive certain moments and I feel myself smile as I smell the sea and I hear laughter.

It is so beautiful outside. We are all at the beach, tanning, chatting and laughing.

I am interrupted by a click as the door slowly opens and the nurse walks in to check my drip.

Day breaks and I must have slept. I have no sense of time anymore. I turn to the chair and mom isn't in it anymore. I face another day; of tests, medication, pain medication and a lumber puncture.

I am transported from one testing section to another, x-rays, C.T scans, sonars. My body aches as they maneuver me into the correct position for the scan. When will it end? Thoughts rush through my mind like wild fire. I know the tests are there to help me with my treatment but don't these people know I am weak and don't feel well.

'Now stay still, don't move and take a deep breath till I say release.'

I take the breath like the lady instructs me to. I close my eyes and pretend I'm somewhere else. My chest aches as I long to release it and breathe normally again.

'Click,' I hear in the background. 'Okay, breathe normally!' she shouts and waits to see if I may have to do it all over again depending on the x-ray image. 'That will be all Chanel' she says. The porter comes to get me and take me back to my room. I am finished until tomorrow I guess.

Mom receives a phone call that Shirley is not coping very well and is on her last. She has already been transferred to the Hospice and is on large doses of morphine for pain and comfort. Mom tells me that she has to leave me here to go and say goodbye to Shirley. She writes me a letter to keep me going until she gets back. I am so selfish, I don't want her to go but I understand that she has to. Aunty Charmaine agrees to come and look after me for the weekend while mom is away. It's weird not having mom here with me, I miss her so much. Aunty Charmaine sits with me and tries to make me smile. I am just too sick to respond. I can't sleep very well and I look out the window and try to think of something nice. My thoughts jump to Shirley and I wonder how she is coping.

Mom says that Shirley changed a lot after she fell ill. She

would hum and moan and look at my mom like she was a stranger. Mom would hold her hand and speak to her saying, 'Mom, I love you.' Shirley would squeeze her hand and mom would know that she was aware of her presence. Shirley was on a permanent morphine drip in the St Francis Hospice in Port Elizabeth. They looked after her very well and when she passed away, mom had peace of mind that she was in good hands.

The funeral was very sad and Shirley was cremated. Mom took her ashes home and they sit next to a photograph of Shirley. I never got to see Shirley after I left for the hospital on the day I was diagnosed but I know that she watches over me every day.

'I love you, Shirley, and I know that we will all see you in heaven again one day.'

Chapter 4

Chemo and the X-block

IT is very traumatic in the x-ray room as I sit and wait for another x-ray to be taken on the hard bed. I look around. Through the window, I see the lady working on the computer. Then another lady walks in and tells me to lie down. I am so thin that the hard surface hurts my bones. I have to be positioned in a very uncomfortable way. She places a hard board over the area they need to take an x-ray of.

'Hold your breath.' She says as she presses the button to take the x-ray.

This is now familiar to me. She then comes in and changes my position. It's exhausting and all I want to do is go back to my room and sleep.

A few days later I have to go through another unbearable bone-marrow biopsy. As with the previous biopsy, I am frightened. The doctor carrying out the biopsy speaks to me, asking me questions about myself to distract and calm me. I see the needle and the feeling of tranquility goes out the window.

First, a tiny prick from an injection filled with local anesthetic to numb the area before they insert the big needle. I feel it going in, it's so painful. It is being twisted and turned in my back hip bone and pressure is applied as if you were opening a wine bottle with a bottle opener. Then comes the pulling. My whole leg goes numb. The pain is excruciating.

Eventually it's over. I lie on my tummy with my arms tucked alongside my body, tears pouring from my eyes and I am shaking. She shows me a tiny glass bottle with the worm-like piece of bone that they have just taken from my hip. It's over and I am taken back to my room to rest.

The next day a lady doctor walks into my room and sits beside my mother and me. She takes my hand and explains to me that the chemo is going to be really harsh on my body and that I will probably not be able to have children one day. The chemo will burn my ovaries and there is generally less than a five percent chance of having a child. At first, I don't fully understand and it doesn't affect me that much.

Mom bursts into tears and takes my hand, turns to me and says, 'My girl, you are so brave. You've already been through so much and now this.'

'It's okay mom, miracles do happen.' My answer puts a smile on her face as we both know that faith and hope are key weapons when fighting any battle.

'It's time to go Chanel,' I am awakened by the sound of my mom's voice which is so reassuring, so gentle. It's time to have my first dose of chemotherapy. This is an anticancer drug that will hopefully stop or at least slow down the growth of the cancer cells in my body.

I have often wondered how she could remain so strong.

The porter is waiting at the door with a wheel chair. Has it really come to this, that I can no longer walk on my own?

I am nauseated at the thought of feeling even more ill. I have been warned about the side-effects of chemotherapy. I climb slowly out of the hospital bed and as I lean forward to take a step, I can feel that my body is not mine anymore. It belongs to this aggressive cancer and I have to fight it. I grip onto mom's arm, she is strong and agile. She knows that I now depend on her completely again. She puts her strong face on and guides me to the wheelchair. I know I am safe in her care.

The porter is a talker, to say the least. Mom makes me giggle as I seep into my chair, listening to how she agrees with everything he is trying to explain to her, is funny to me. Mom always tries to make people feel important. She would never tell him to stop talking. That's just how she is, completely selfless. Down we go in the lift to the ground floor, through a dark passage, into a tunnel and down, down, down we go towards X-Block. I'm afraid now, not knowing is the worst feeling I think. As we slowly approach the end of the tunnel I start feeling nervous.

At the door, we are warmly greeted by the sweetest female nurse. The room has pretty, floral, yellow curtains. The chairs are all different styles of lazy boys, comfy and safe and it is nothing like I expected after going through all those dark places to get here. It seems similar to my journey with this illness. At that moment I had a realisation; there is light at the end of the tunnel. I am safe in God's care and these people are here to assist in God's glorious plan. My mom looks around and finds me a comfortable chair in the corner. As the porter leaves and says goodbye, I sit back in my chair.

The sister (head nurse) talks me through what is going to happen. *Then the fear comes again.* I hate needles. I cannot stand that feeling but I know it has to be done. Mom holds my hand as a tear drops down my cheek. The sister takes my hand and checks for a vein. She wipes my hand with an alcohol swab. She takes the needle from the protective packet and says, 'This is going to sting.' The needle goes into my vein, then the sister pulls out the silver sharp bit and the white plastic tube stays behind in my hand. It is then connected to my drip. It isn't even that painful I think to myself until she puts up the chemo bag. Mom and I both look up at it. As the first drop flows through the pipe and into my veins I start to shout a bit, 'Ouch! It burns, take it out! Take it out!'

Mom squeezes my hand. I am crying now but I'm surrounded by people who are in the same position as me and I can see how they are all staring at me. This is something I need to do to survive. I should stop being such a baby and take this pain. The sister comes with an injection and injects me in the arm to calm me and relieve some of the pain. People start to communicate with us and conversation breaks out in the room.

I am feeling hungry, which is a great sign. Mom is pleased to hear that I have an appetite. I look at the window as the sun hits the window pane. It truly is beautiful. I think to myself: *this journey is long but I know that I will fight and get to the end of it.*

The last drop goes into my hand. The burning sensation was so consistent throughout the chemo session that I feel as though my hand is numb. The sister disconnects the drip and screws a lid onto the apparatus of the needle in my hand.

'This needle can stay in your hand for now, so that they don't have to prick you again later,' she says with a soft gentle smile.

Dr. Els walks into the room and says. 'Hello Chanel. Unfortunately, we are going to have to do a lumber puncture on you now'.

Oh no! That's terrible. After this pain, here comes more. I sit up on the bed and the curtains are closed around me. I grip my mom's hand again. First, Dr. Els injects me with a local anesthetic through the needle in my hand. This is followed by a sedative shot and then comes the long needle. It is inserted into my middle back spinal cord and fluid is extracted. This fluid must be tested to determine whether the cancer has spread to my brain.

I wake up a few minutes later with a dressing on my back and a bad headache, not to mention the pain. To my surprise Dr. Els and my mom are laughing. Now this is new.

'What are you laughing at?' I ask.

'Couldn't you choose someone better than Chuck Norris, Chanel?' Replies Dr. Els.

'Ha ha ha ha. Umm, what are you guys talking about?'

It turns out that while I was sedated with dormicum (a drug that makes you forget about the procedure but can still feel everything throughout the procedure) I was flirting with Chuck Norris, in my sedated state. Okay, that was funny.

I am so exhausted now and the porter is waiting to take me back to my room. I begin to feel the effects of the chemo. It's extreme nausea. Dr. Schmidt is waiting in my room and gives me an anti-nausea shot into my saline drip. He also gives me a shot of morphine for the pain. The minute it enters my body I throw up. It feels terrible. I lie down and my eyelids begin to get heavy. I fall asleep. This becomes routine for me. I have chemo, get the anti-nausea and pain meds, throw up and fall asleep. I was eventually on five millimetres of morphine every four hours.

I am told that I will need to have a J-line inserted as the

chemo sessions get more frequent. This is a catheter that is surgically inserted into your neck vein and attached to your collar bone cartilage and then the other side is threaded out from your chest. At the end of the catheter there is a two-way pipe; one for blood transfusions and medication and the other for chemotherapy. This will ensure that I will not have to be pricked all the time. Not only is it painful to constantly have a needle jabbed into you but it causes severe bruising and could cause blood clots. The J-line is a safer and more effective solution. Dad comes to Cape Town to be with us for this procedure. When they wheel me into the operating room, my mom and dad wait for me in the waiting room. I am so scared. I don't know what is going to happen. The anesthetist puts the mask over my face and asks me to count backwards from ten. He then injects a yellowish solution into my drip and I start to count. *10, 9, 8...* and then I wake up and see my parents.

'She's awake.' I try to turn towards them but my neck is stiff and painful. It feels so weird and I am convinced that my J-line has been inserted incorrectly. I get up after the anesthetic wears off but I cannot move my neck properly. Mom and dad find this very funny. Now, looking back, so do I.

The chemo in the X-Block seems like a breeze now. I am not scared anymore because I know what to expect, plus I have my new J-line and don't have to deal with needles anymore. Mom is more relaxed as she can see how I have progressed from when I first started. I am more relaxed and even start making friends in the X-Block.

One family we met was a mother and her son who was around my age. He would talk to me and tell me what to expect. My mom and his mom would chat about us and what they were going through. They even brought us home-cooked meals in hospital. It was great to have their support.

Then we hear even greater news. At the beginning of my treatment I was told that I would need a bone marrow transplant so both my brothers were tested. The donor should preferably be a sibling or by some luck a cousin and it cannot be your parents. We were hoping and praying that the results would come back and one of my brothers would be a positive match. We would have to continue our search overseas if the results were negative.

We would need a lot of money to be able to search for a suitable donor. Dad was in Port Elizabeth with Sheldon and Daine to do the tests. Now, months later, as mom and I are sitting in the X-Block for my chemo treatment, Doctor Schmidt walks in and tells my mom he has some great news for us, 'Daine is a 99.9 percent match. Wow!' This is the greatest news ever. Mom bursts into tears and we all are so happy. Mom calls dad immediately to share the news. I have to wait until I am in full remission before I can have my transplant.

Tests follow throughout the year. The C.T. scan is the most horrible test for me as I am claustrophobic. They inject this ink-like liquid into my drip. I can almost taste it, it's so strong. The C.T. scan is to check inside my body, the blood vessels, muscle tissue, internal organs, bones, basically everything. The liquid makes all these things show up on a screen. The machine is like a tunnel and I am placed on the movable bed and wheeled in and out of the tunnel as the pictures are taken. I have to keep extremely still and relax. It's hard for me. I close my eyes as my heart beats faster. This is a nightmare. I start to scream. Mom rushes to me and holds my hand.

'I want to get out.' I scream.

The doctors eventually have to give me a sedative to calm me down. I lie there crying, my body and mind numb.

This is all for my own good but does it have to be so painful and uncomfortable.

They finally finish and I am so relieved. I start to feel nauseous as mom helps me off the bed. I am still a bit dizzy and all I want is to go back to my room and sleep.

The days are dragging and I have to endure all these things and still come out on top. It's really hard. It's not something I would wish on my worst enemy. Most of my days are spent thinking. I even start writing a diary but it isn't long before I can no longer even hold a pen. As my body grows weaker, so does my mind and my faith. I fight hard but at the same time a little thing in my mind is telling me to just give up. I have to face my deepest fears I feel I was just thrown in and told to swim. Sometimes the water seems too deep but there is always a life jacket for me and at the end of the water, the lifeguard.

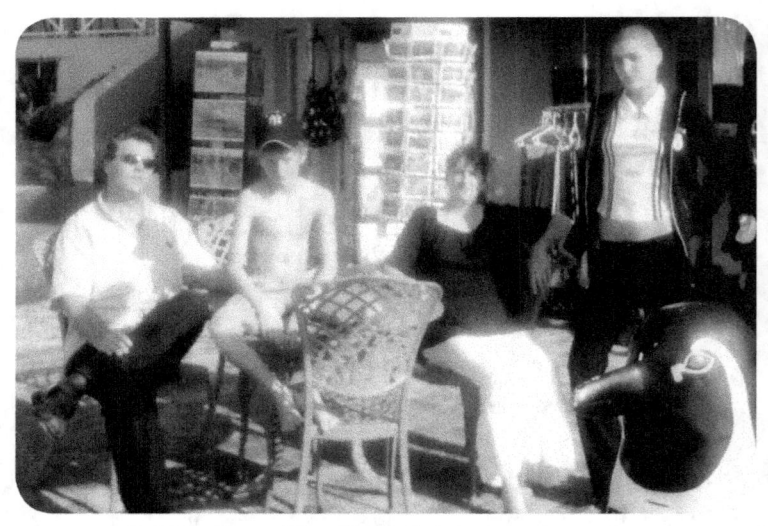

Dad, Daine, Mom and Chanel, in Cape Town, just before the transplant

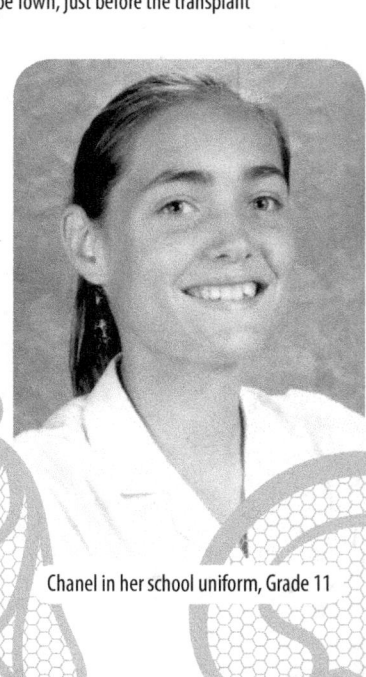

Chanel in her school uniform, Grade 11

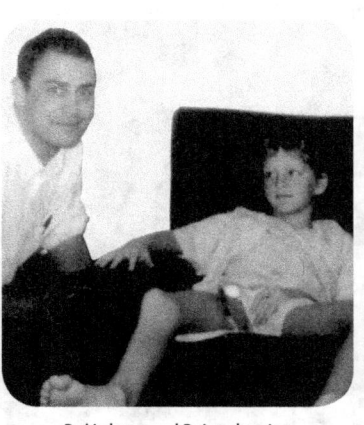

Dr Littleton and Daine showing
the post in his groin

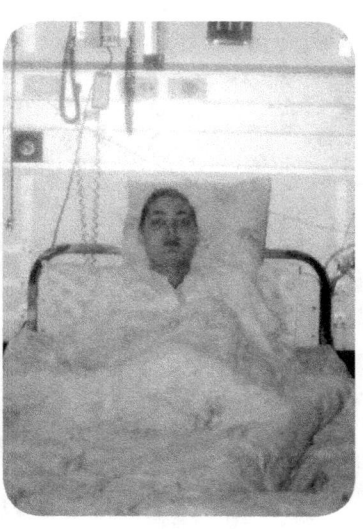

Chanel in hospital

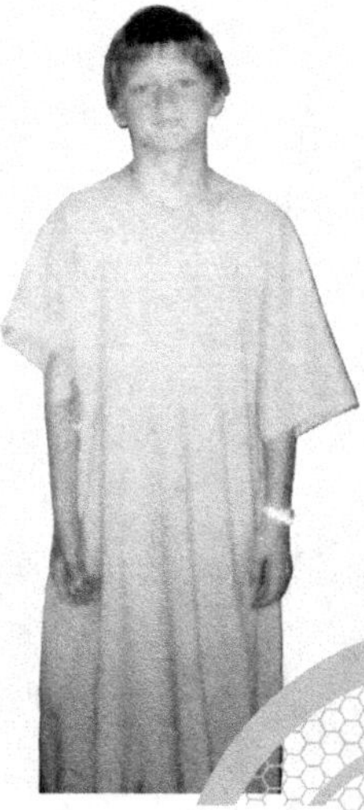

Daine in his hospital gown

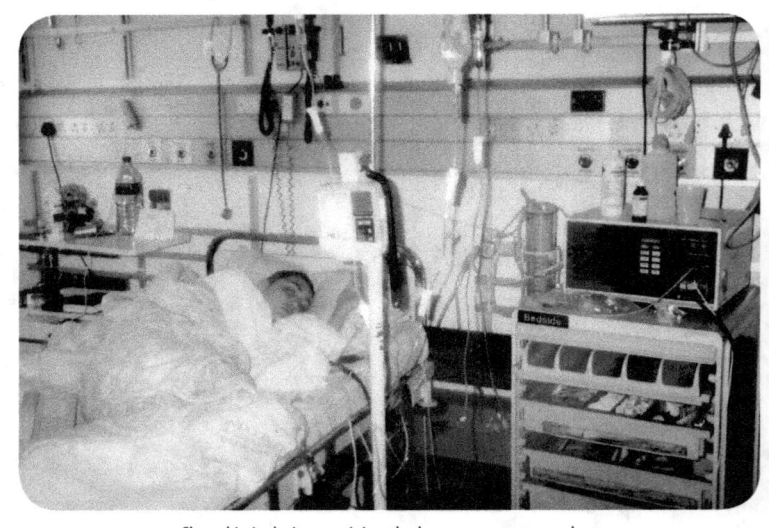

Chanel in isolation receiving the bone-marrow transplant

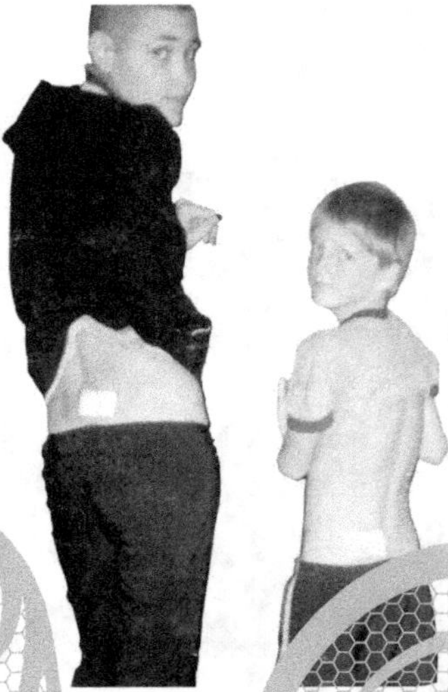

Chanel and Daine after the
bone-marrow transplant

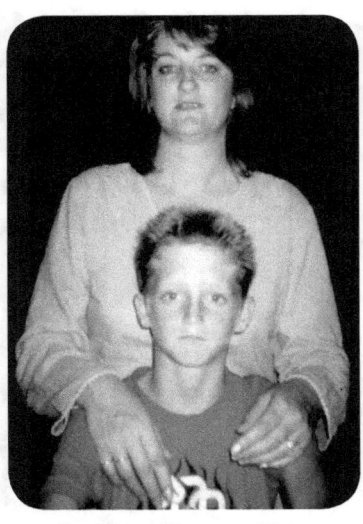

Mom, Shireen Wewege, and Daine

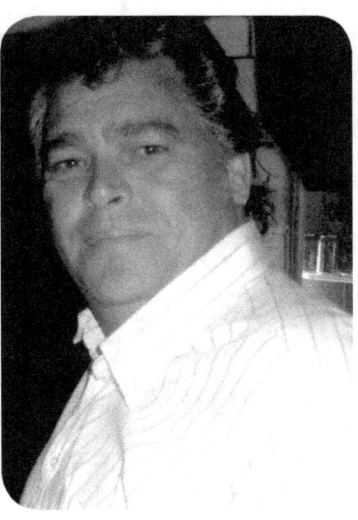

Dad, Johhny Wewege

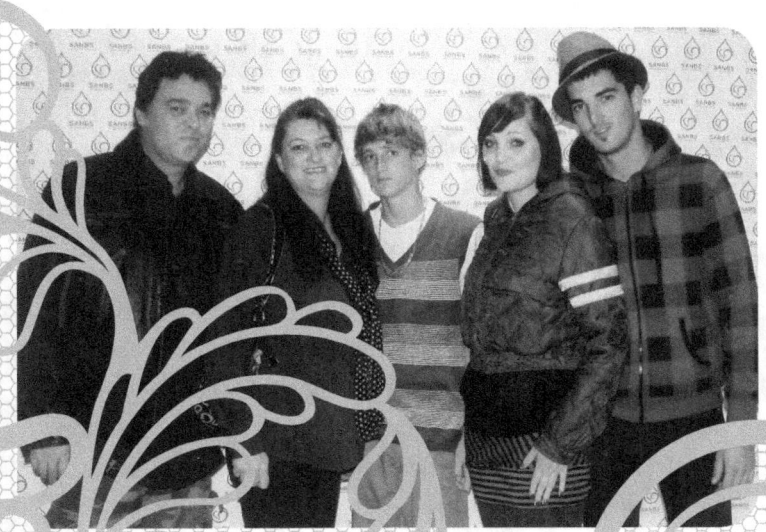

Dad, Mom, Daine, Chanel and Sheldon

Chapter 5

Losing more than my hair

One of the most traumatic experiences for me was losing my hair. Just saying it doesn't really make an impact, but when you go through it, you lose more than just your hair.

I knew it was going to happen, the doctors explained it to me. I guess I just don't want to accept it. When your hair starts falling out, it means that the chemo is working its' way through your body and killing off your cells. It makes you realise that what's happening is real. It starts off slowly. I wake up with little bits of hair on my pillow. I am developing a huge knot in my hair from lying down all the time. I won't let mom brush my hair, it's too sore. Dad calls it a huge dreadlock. It looks like a beehive. When I try to untangle it, it just gets worse.

One of my nurses is a beautiful foreign lady. She is tiny, has really dark skin, is in her mid-thirties and has a big heart. I actually start crying when she enters my room. She really makes an entrance. She comes in singing and dancing, opens my curtains, asks me how I am feeling and tells me what a beautiful day it is outside. Then she takes a brush and tries to untangle my hair. It hurts and irritates me. I start to scream because the more she brushes it, the more pieces of my hair stay behind on the brush. I am a real brat I think because when I look back, she was just trying to keep me positive.

She then decides to cream my entire body with body lotion while I am kicking and screaming. I beg my mom to make her stop. She just ignores my pleas and starts telling me how she and I are going to run on the beach soon and play in the water. This makes me even more agitated as I have finally started to accept that I am sick and now this lady is giving me false hope.

Now I know that her words of encouragement were actually penetrating my mind without me realising it. She sings gospel songs and has the most beautiful voice, like an angel. Mom likes her singing. So do I, deep down inside. *I wish that I could remember her name and all the others too. These are the people I would like to thank personally, the people who made a huge impact in my life.*

The hair on my pillow is increasing by the day, so hospital volunteer hair-dressers are called in. They wash my hair; half dry it with a towel and then proceed to cut it. It's hard for me to let go, but if they don't cut it, it will be even more difficult for me when it falls out in big chunks. The lady tries her best to make it look good but I'm too sad to even bother looking. The day is very hard for me. I'm really quiet and I just do whatever I have to do and take whatever medication is needed to get through the day. The chemo is taking its toll on me and my body is deteriorating at a rapid rate. My hair falls out completely. Every time the nurses or doctors walk into my room I grab my blanket and put it over my head. I start screaming for them to go away because I don't want them to see me like this. It is mentally draining. I get some bandanas to wear from the sunflower foundation. I don't even know how to wear a bandana with no hair underneath it. I eventually learn and time heals that episode. I get used to the fact that my hair is gone.

Mom helps to bath and dress me. I am reduced to being fully dependent on her. I can't even walk on my own anymore. Mom holds me by the arm and the two of us walk up and down the passage, past all the other rooms in the cancer ward greeting the nurses along the way. The passage is only about ten metres long from my room to the waiting area but to me it feels as though I've been walking for ten kilometres. When we get to the end, I have to sit and rest for a while before going back. I am just skin and bones and weigh no more than 35 to 40 kilograms. My height is 1.78 metres so I know I must look dreadful. We go back to my room and I lie down. I promise myself that I will not look in a mirror. I don't want to see what I've become.

One night mom is bathing me and as I step up to get out, holding tight onto mom's arm to get my balance, I accidentally catch a glimpse of myself in the small mirror of the medicine cabinet. I stand still and stare at myself in shock. I look at my mom and we both start crying. She tells me it won't always be like this, I'm going to get better. I look like a ghost, my cheek bones stick out from my face and my eyes are sunken. My J-line pipe is hanging from my body and I can see my ribs clearly. I am a skeleton. I have little patches of hair on my head. I don't recognise myself and I'm really scared.

Mom takes me back to my bed and I crawl to it. My drip stand is packed with different drips as well as a heart monitor. I am getting used to the five millimetres of morphine every four hours and my body is weak. I am not allowed to eat any food from outside the hospital and a dietician is assigned to create the meals that I am allowed to have. I'm craving for a hamburger, pasta, anything that isn't hospital food. My skin is discoloured and appears blotchy and darker. I am transforming into a different person altogether and there is nothing I can do to stop it.

Every day is a battle, I am no longer able to go to the X-Block for my chemo as I am so weak and it now has to be administered in my room while I lie in bed. I remember the taste of the chemo. There are different types of chemotherapy some stronger than others. It tastes like metal as it drips into my veins and is extremely unpleasant. Sometimes I just lie there and cry and other times I just hold mom's hand and we talk through it. The best times are when I fall asleep and wake up and find it's finished. Unfortunately, every time the chemo is finished the painful cramps in my tummy start and I am given my morphine shot which will make me throw up again. I almost give up my fight but mom guides me to continue fighting. One type of chemo has to be covered with a bag because it can explode if exposed to the sun. It is a petroleum reddish colour. My heart is getting weaker and weaker as I lie in hospital. I have to have regular blood transfusions to keep my red blood count stable. I acknowledge that I am going through the hardest thing I have ever experienced in my life and all I can do is pray and hope for the best.

Dad comes to visit every now and then and these visits are the highlight of our year. When he walks into the room we feel instantly happier. I sit with my Walkman earphones and play my Evanescence CD. I love to sing. I learn all the Evanescence songs in that year and I sit on my bed singing them. One day I was facing the wall, sitting with my back to the door. Mom and dad went for a walk and when they returned they walked into my room. I didn't hear them. I was singing. When I reached the end of the song I turned around and they were both crying. 'What's wrong'? I ask. They say I sing like an angel. I just smile.

I turn 18 years of age in hospital on the 10 June 2004. It's not much of a birthday but at least I have one. Mom, dad, Daine and Sheldon are here and we ask the doctors if we can go out for something to eat to celebrate my birthday. The chemo is working and the cancer is under control. I am slowly but surely building up strength again so we are given permission to go out. A curfew is given and we're told to stick to it. I am in the early stages of remission which means that my immune system is still very low and if I catch any sort of germ, I could be in great danger and the complications could be fatal. This is explained to us very thoroughly by doctor's Els and Schmidt before we are released. We go to the Spur in the Tygerburg area for some lunch. As we walk in, everyone looks at us. There are people staring at us from all angles. This angers and saddens me all at the same time. I look at them and even comment that they have no shame. I tell them to stop looking at me. Mom and dad calm me down and take me to the table.

I order a hamburger, something I had been longing for. I eat a bit and lie down. It is an exhausting task just to eat. We ask someone to take a photo of us. It is a lovely family outing. I get tired very quickly, so after our meal we head back to the hospital. Looking back at that photo, I am reminded of how sick I really was. We are a little bit late getting back but Dr. Els forgives us. It's so nice just to spend time with my family. Dad and the boys have to go back. Dad has to start work on Monday and the boys have to go back to school. Mom and I dread it when they have to leave.

We go back to our usual daily routine. Tygerburg is a training hospital so I am introduced to some students who will take my blood and study me. I find this so weird but at least I can aid in them in becoming doctors one day. One morning, a student is taking blood from my J-line and ends up blocking one of the tubes. The doctors are so angry with him. This is bad news for me because if the remaining tube gets blocked up from overuse I will have to have another J-line put in and there could be complications. Thankfully the other one continued to work just fine. It's nice when the students come to visit. They're always so enthusiastic and I can see that they are becoming fond of me. There is a friendship growing. They talk to me and ask how I am feeling. Just to have some form of the outside world in my room is wonderful for me because I feel so disconnected at times.

Chapter 6

Too close for comfort

I have reached the point where I am too weak to go to the toilet. The doctors tell mom and me that I have to have a catheter. This is a bag that helps your bladder to work without you having to do anything; basically you cannot even feel yourself urinate. At one point I had to wear nappies which were really terrible for me, degrading and embarrassing. Fortunately, it wasn't for too long as I regained my strength day by day.

One day I started to swell up and my skin has a yellowish tinge. My breathing becomes faster and I am gasping for air. My body is unrecognisable and my ankles swell up to the size of my thighs. I have developed a yellow jaundice infection due to my liver taking so much strain from the chemo and medication. I am told to drink a special mixture from the dietician in an attempt to revive my liver. It's really a tasty lime mixture which I must drink once a day.

I am put on an oxygen mask to aid my breathing. One day, as I am sitting in bed reading with the oxygen mask on, I just start to feel strange. I feel as if I am suffocating. I signal to my mom that I can't breathe because I can't talk either and then I hear a loud beep as my heart monitor signals a problem. The nurses and doctors come rushing in and all of a sudden a six-inch needle gets inserted into my lung, between my rib cage to suck out an air bubble. An air bubble has formed in my drip and if not caught in time I could have died right then.

The shock of that moment makes me realise that this is no joke. I am hanging on by a thread. There is no guarantee that I will even make it through another day. Eventually the yellow jaundice goes away and I am slowly improving. I start to get these weird cold attacks where I shiver for hours and the nurses' pile on blankets to try and soothe me. There is nothing else they can do. I can't talk either as my teeth are shaking or rattling. Eventually they subside and I pass out from exhaustion. Mom is so frightened all the time. Every time something happens she calls my dad.

The days continue bringing new fears. I start getting really severe tummy pains and it comes to the point where I need to have pethadene or morphine every day depending on the intensity of the pain, five millimetres every four hours. My body is becoming immune to morphine so I need something that works faster and is stronger. My colon has torn. This is not good news. The pain is excruciating. I feel like I am being stabbed in the stomach over and over again. My stools become a pitch black liquid and I am unable to eat or drink anything for the next month. I am put on a drip containing nutrients and I am only permitted to suck ice to quench my thirst.

I lie in agony and discomfort. Dad and the boys come to visit often and I am always so happy to see them. Mom chats to dad about everything that happens in the hospital while he is away. My brothers, Sheldon and Daine, hang around my bedside and watch TV in my room. I am starving but cannot eat. I am thirsty but cannot drink. It's torture. Dad and mom have a Fanta Grape and I long to have just one sip. Dad cannot stand to see me suffer so he sneaks a few drops in a cup and I drink it. It tastes so great, the best I have ever had. I want more but I know I can't have any.

I immediately get the most terrible cramps in my tummy. I scream in pain. It is excruciating. The nurse runs in to see what has happened and it is revealed that I had drunk a little cold drink. I had caused my own complications. This means that I will now go for a few more days without food and water. Every morning Dr. Els collects a stool sample. It is still black. Only when the colour changes will I be allowed to eat solids and drink again. I suffer for a few more weeks until the sample is eventually approved. I remember being so happy.

To prevent any unnecessary germs I have to be in semi-isolation. I feel scared to face the outside world again as I have grown attached to this lifestyle now. I pray every night and as letters and prayers come streaming in I at least feel some connection to life. Mom and I watch TV and play games to pass the long days and nights.

One particular evening we're not in the mood for hospital food again. We get a Mr. Delivery booklet and start looking through it for something nice to eat. I feel like a hamburger. Mom spots an interesting looking advert for an American burger place. She calls and places an order for two. We patiently wait for our meal to arrive. Mom and I open our polystyrene boxes and to our surprise the hamburger is the size of a pizza. It was the hugest burger I had ever seen. I couldn't even open my mouth wide enough to take a bite. We laugh about the fact that we couldn't even eat half of that hamburger, it was so massive. We laugh so much that the tears pour out of our eyes. It's the first time in a long time that we laugh like this. We get tired and fall asleep talking.

Being in hospital so long and having mom by my side each and every day helps us to develop an even stronger bond and we now rely on each other to get through the year. The time for my transplant is approaching and I am excited and terribly nervous. My medication intake is increasing and the chemotherapy is harsh. The test results show that I am in the early stages of remission and that my blood count is improving daily. Every day we pray. There are people all over South Africa praying, maybe even the world. It is truly remarkable how powerful prayer is.

The hospital is getting expensive. My dad and the boys are constantly travelling up and down from Port Elizabeth to Cape Town and the cost of food and toiletries is getting too much for us to handle on top of everything else. My parents' friends Michael and Mandy organise a Golf Day in order to raise funds and awareness for me. There are t-shirts made with my name on the sleeve that read: Chanel Wewege 2004. Maybe you know someone who has one, now you know why. Aunty Jean and the ladies in my family are organising an auction to raise funds too. The support is overwhelming and each day is a blessing.

Reach for a Dream is coming by to ask me what my dream is. I think of my brothers as I stare at the sheet of paper in front of me asking me to state my dream. I want them to be happy too, so I ask for a Sony Play Station. *The Reach for a Dream* programme is a very worthy cause because hospital tends to make you forget you are still young and there is a whole world outside these walls that we should be a part of too. The *Sunflower Association* for Leukemia patients gave me bandanas to wear so that my head was always covered in one of their brightly coloured designs. A number of companies are trying to make life a little bit easier for children and teenagers living with cancer. We are still children, we still want to play and we still need to dream even though we are going through a painful journey.

The *CHOC Childhood Cancer Foundation* made it possible to still be in a normal environment with our families during this difficult time. All of you are special. God puts people like you on this earth to help us get through the pain and struggles we face. Many times my status was not looking good and more and more prayers were circulating. I always kept 'hope' close by and recognised God's blessings. Even if I didn't make it, at least I knew I would be in paradise and without pain one day.

I lie in bed here in hospital thinking about how my life used to be. I would sleep over at my cousins place and we would warm up hotdogs in the microwave in the middle of the night, after coming home from an under 18's party. We would tip-toe and try not to make a noise. Aunty Jean would wake up and come and chat to us about our evening. Those were such special times. I think about how I would come home from school on a Friday and smell Shirley in the doorway and I just knew that she would be sitting on the couch chatting away to my mom who would be in the kitchen. I would run and give her a big hug and a kiss. These memories make me smile and I long to have those times back again. I share many hours with God and I speak to Him all the time. I say to God that if He heals me, I will spread the word of His miracles and I will make a difference.

I also have terrible thoughts about death. Many nights I have bad dreams of fire and pain. I am so confused but I keep my faith. Although it gets very difficult sometimes and I am extremely weak, I always manage to get up again. It is a tough choice to make, life or death.

The time had eventually arrived for me to go home for a month, before my transplant. Mom and I are so excited. I was also sad to leave as Tygerburg F10 had become my home. The nurses and doctors had become my family. I suppose I am afraid of the unknown and for everyone to see me like this. I weigh almost nothing and I cannot stand up on my own. I have to be transported to the plane in a wheelchair. I'm almost frightened to be outside these walls. Mom wanted to organise all my friends to be waiting for me at the airport but I begged her not to. I don't want them to see me like this.

Chapter 7

Home for a while

I'M carried by my mom and an airport helper to my wheelchair and wheeled into the luggage section at the airport. It's so good to be back in Port Elizabeth and to be outside. My eyes hurt from the bright light and I know that people are staring at me from all directions. Eventually, mom and I get our luggage and we see everyone waiting for us through the glass; dad, Daine, Sheldon, Eve (my grandmother from my dad's side), my cousins, Chavonne, Shannon, Merle and Aunty Jean. They all come running to greet us. They hesitate for a moment and Hannah, my baby cousin is not sure who I am. That hurts, but I know I will be back to the way I was really soon. They wheel me to the parking lot and I can see how happy mom is to be home again.

As we drive up to our house we notice a lot changes and the house is a different colour on the outside. Maybe I'm imagining it as we have been away for so long. As we make our way towards the front door, surprise! The whole house has been renovated. The entire family got together and everyone did their bit to redecorate the house. My bedroom had been transformed into a beautiful tranquil space with dolphin decorations on my bedding and curtains, plus a new bed. The carpets had been removed and the old wooden floors that were underneath them had been sanded and newly varnished. It was a great surprise and mom was over the moon. Somehow though, I longed for it to be how it was. I needed 'my' home. It smelt different too. I felt like I was walking into a foreign room but I was happy that my parents were happy.

The first thing I want is roast potatoes, Aunty Jean's roast potatoes. I had been craving them and with my appetite back, I knew I had to take advantage of it. She makes a few for me and I happily eat them in my new bed. Later, everyone comes to visit and it's an exhausting night. Everyone is asking questions and all I want to do is to sleep. Eventually everyone leaves and I'm left with hugs and kisses from mom and dad once again.

I now have a collection of teddy bears from different people who sent them to me while I was in hospital. I stare at them for a while. I am still extremely weak and mom still helps me to bath. The days leading up to my transplant are spent mostly with my family. I feel afraid as I know that there could be complications and the chances of my body rejecting the new bone-marrow are a lot greater than I am comfortable with. I was given a whole bag of medication to take while at home. I have to make sure I stay as healthy as possible before the transplant. I keep myself positive and pray all the time.

I want to be myself again. I want the transplant to be over and done with so that I can move on with my life. I am strictly prohibited from going to any crowded areas like shopping malls and restaurants, anywhere where there are a lot of people. This is because my immune system is so low that if I pick up any type of germ I could become severely ill. And this would mean the end of me and my battle with cancer.

I sit in bed most of the time reading and writing. Mom encourages me to get up and sit outside and get some fresh air. I am so tired but I force myself to get up. Today I am going to spend time with my cousins. I get there and everything seems different. I hold onto the wall and make my way inside. It's so weird, these are the girls I grew up with and we literally did everything together, now I feel like an outsider. They try to understand that I can no longer do what we used to do. I think it's tough for all of us. They make me a sandwich and we sit by the pool. Soon, it's time to go home as I'm starting to get drowsy again.

My J-line is still in and the bandage has to be changed every few days. It's really painful when the nurses change the dressing so I am very nervous about mom doing it for me. Reluctantly, she gently pulls off the see-through sticker-like dressing away from my skin. Everything is fine until she gets to the actual entrance wound that the line is coming out of. I screech as she gently tries to remove the dressing. Mom takes out an alcohol swab in order to clean it, wiping gently and making sure I'm not watching. She then puts the new dressing on and I sigh with relief. I look at myself in the mirror, my ribs stick out and my J-line hangs from my neck. I wear a wig to cover my bald head. I feel emotionally drained.

My Business Economics teacher Mrs. Blignaud, from Pearson High and two of my friends from school, Wayne Wilson and Shanna Harth come to visit me. I immediately and apologetically want to hide myself. They reassure me that it's all fine and I sit down and listen to them talk about everything and its really great having them here. Otherwise, I spend as much time as possible with dad and the boys. The time for the transplant is fast approaching and before we know it, the dates are set and the doctors are ready for me at Groote Schuur Hospital.

Chapter 8

The transplant

A few days before I go into complete isolation, Daine and I have to have a bone-marrow biopsy. I am familiar with the procedure and so I dread it for my little brother. Mom, Dad, Daine and I walk into the Groote Schuur Cancer Hematology clinic. This is where all the procedures are carried out. The waiting room is full of people who have cancer and are fighting for their lives.

Daine is given a sedative pill called Dormicum. The same medication I was given in Tygerburg but in tablet form, as he is too young to have the injection. This tablet is very strong and we are told that it will start working in about twenty minutes. Dad and mom go out for a cigarette and Daine tags along. A few minutes later dad walks in carrying Daine as he cannot stand and his legs are like jelly. He starts talking in a funny way and his eyes are rolling back. The nurses rush to put him on a bed. Dad starts to panic and mom starts to cry. 'It's all normal,' says the doctor. Daine lies on the bed and stares at us as he is wheeled into the procedure room.

He starts to sing. 'Two trailer park girls go round the outside. Guess who's back, back again!' Everyone starts laughing as he is singing really loudly. The doctors and my parents wheel him into the surgical room. I sit in the waiting room. They tell him they are going to insert the needle and then he starts screaming. Saliva is drooling from his mouth as he screams in agony.

I start to shake and my body feels his pain. Daine was in so much pain, that my dad had to hold his head down as he kept on jumping up. Luckily, it didn't take that long and he came out crying and holding my dad's hand. He fell asleep a few minutes later. It's my turn. I get onto the bed and I tell the doctor what's going to happen before he can even start to tell me. I suppose my fear was making me so talkative. He and the nurse smile at me. The procedure starts with the local anesthetic, then the Dormicum and finally the big needle. I grind my teeth as it enters my skin and then my bone and then came the jerk and it was all over. They hold up the test tube and show me the piece of bone as they bandage the wound.

I am wheeled into the same room as my brother. He is still under sedation and mom says she is worried that he will never come right and starts to cry again. I put my face close to him and he punched me square in the face. (Yes, I got that line from the movie: 'Step Brother'). We all start laughing. Another thing to remember when going through something like this, watch funny movies and laugh. We both fall asleep and when we wake up Daine can't remember a thing.

It's the last night that I will be free for a while as I will have to be in strict isolation.

The next day we all went to the hospital to settle me in. My room, F6, was small but cozy. There was an en-suite bathroom and big windows. It had two separate entrances and in between the two doorways stood a basin and a bar of soap. I would have to be in complete isolation before, during and after the transplant. The year was almost over and my battle with cancer would hopefully soon be over and I could start to live a normal life again.

My room was to be my new 'home'. My heart began to beat faster and faster as I begin to feel claustrophobic. I thought I have to do this – I have come so far already. Daine and dad are ready to leave again. Mom will have to stay at the Kerkhuis alone. Mom stayed with me till night fell. We joked around as I settled in, thinking it couldn't be that bad. I had already experienced such a lot, how could this be worse. I'm given a blood transfusion and some other medication via a drip. I'm told that I will have to undergo chemotherapy again. I am familiar with how it will make me feel and a tear falls from my cheek onto my lap.

Dr. Neil Littleton is my new doctor. We had heard great things about him which turn out to be true. We are taken to a small office to meet him. We listen as he tells us that there are no guarantees and the chances of survival are 50/50... He also tells us that if the transplant is not successful there is no way we can try again as my heart would be too weak to withstand it. This news hit me like a bus and I sat back in the chair and just stared at him. Mom started to cry but she knew she had to be strong. There were no certainties from the beginning and we just had to take one day at a time.

I had brought my sound system with me and Evanescence was right there in my CD player. She kept me going as did God, my parents, brothers, family, and friends. I must admit, some friends kept their distance. I suppose it was due to their fear of not knowing how to handle the situation. All the support I had kept me sane.

My medication increased and I had to swallow a lot of tiny, yellow, oral chemo tablets as well as a whole bunch of other pills. I am put on supplement called Ensure to help me keep my strength up. Every morning when I stand on the scale I weigh less and less. I try to drink the Ensure but I get nauseous and throw it up most of the time. The chemo starts taking its toll. I'm losing weight dramatically and everyone is worried about me. Tests and bone-marrow biopsies are looming again and I dread every second. I look out of the window and watch the people as they walk up and down the streets. I long to be outside, to be like them – to be normal. The blinds continually hits against the window pane.

I can still remember that sound.

Mom stays with me throughout the day and at the Kerkhuis in the evening. It is a guest house for people in hospital. It is walking distance from Groote Schuur Hospital and the people who work there are kind and helpful. Mom is not allowed to be by my side when I sleep. No germs are allowed to enter my new domain. I am completely isolated and forbidden to leave my room. I feel like I am in prison, serving a sentence.

I wake up to the sound of the nurse entering my room in order to change my bedding, weigh me and take my temperature. Each day they replace the un-touched Ensure bottle with a new one. I also have to drink sterilised water as the tap water could infect me with parasites. It tastes like medicine. After the doctors rounds are over I wait patiently for mom to arrive. She comes in wearing a blue surgical outfit, booties and all. She has to wash her hands twice before entering my room. A maximum of two visitors are permitted at a time. I'm so happy to see her.

This routine goes on for days until Daine and dad come up for the stem cell procedure. The nurse comes in with my chemo bag for the day. It is neon red in colour, like petrol. I know how it's going to make me feel. This is the most important chemo, the strongest dosage to kill all my cells before the transplant to make way for the new stem cells. I only manage to eat little bits of my food. Every morning the doctors come and see me. They ask me how I am feeling and talk about me as if I am not there. I am very despondent and in pain I try to be a 'good patient,' but because I'm so uncomfortable, I make them suffer with me.

One morning, Dr. Littleton walks in on his daily rounds to check up on me, along with the rest of his patients. I'm in pain and cry out to him that my tummy is really sore and that I'm so thin and how much I hate it. He looks at me and says, 'Chanel, do you know how many girls would die to look like you right now?' I am speechless. He is straight forward and honest and always has a positive thing to say that will brighten up even your darkest day.

The days drag by and my drip stand becomes heavier as my medication increases. I get up to shower in the mornings. The shower curtain has a gap in it for the drip's pipes. I shower carefully not to wet my J-line too much. I am unable to stand up straight as my stomach has sunken inwards and I am weak and nauseous all the time. I have a permanent morphine drip now which consists of saline mixed with morphine. I am also attached to a heart monitor. Every day seems like it will never end. The time drags as I try to entertain myself drawing and writing. I am often too sick to even get up. Mom is lonely. She stays with me for most of the day and then has to return to the Kerkhuis when evening falls. Mom tells me about the people in the Kerkhuis and how I would love them and they would really like me she says. I long for the day that I will be out of this hospital. I've spent almost a month in isolation.

Dad arrives in Cape Town for a short visit. Mom shows dad how to enter the room. Dad seems distant; I can see that it's strange for him to see me like this. Mom is used to it but dad is deeply moved. Every now and then he has a tear in his eye – he was probably remembering how I used to look. One evening he wrote a poem for me on a piece of paper. It was something he had read that reminded him of me. It was a wonderful piece. I misplaced that little piece of paper; little did I know how utterly significant it would be to me today! Dad went home filled with sadness and pain in his heart after seeing me go through this isolation period and having to leave his wife behind. Days passed like months as we tried to keep each other sane. The only thing that kept us going was prayer, love and laughter.

The time has finally arrived to fetch Daine for the transplant. Mom went home to PE to fetch him. It was a long, miserable three days without her.

Mom and Daine arrive in Cape Town. Mom walks in and hugs me. I see Daine peeping through the glass as no children are allowed inside my room. He put his little hands up against the window and peered in then waved hysterically at me. My heart sank. He was here, ready for battle. That evening he had to start the cell boosting injections he was to have for the next three days. Mom had to inject him in his thigh every four hours during the night. She said that it was very painful for him as it burnt. She hated to put him through that pain but he was adamant that he wanted to save his sister. These injections were to prepare his stem cells for the transplant. It was so good to have him near, even though I couldn't touch his little hands.

The day for my transplant finally dawned. Daine was

taken to a hospital room in the pediatric ward. Mom bought him Nik-Naks, chocolate and a cool drink. The process Daine underwent is called Apheresis; the peripheral blood stem cell collection process in which blood is taken from one patient and circulated through a machine that separates out stem cells. The remaining cells are then returned to the patient. This would take a while to complete. Daine was not allowed to move out of the bed once connected to the machine. He was taken to an operating room where Dr Littleton surgically inserted a port into his groin under general anesthetic. When it was over, he woke up screaming in pain.

'It really burns, hey, mom,' he said with red eyes.

He was still very drowsy and was told to rest for a while. When he woke up again, he was taken to the room where the stem cell machine was. Mom sat next to him during most of the process, held his hand and said she was so sorry he had to go through this pain. He said, *'But you know what, Mom, I would do it all again to save my sister's life.'*

Mom said she would never forget those words from her nine year old son. Mom ran between him and me to check up on both of us. Daine spent the time watching cartoons and he said it wasn't bad sitting there for hours.

On the other side of the hospital I am busy preparing myself for the transplant. I am scared. I know this could be the end of the cancer or the end of my life. The nurse comes in and gives me a pre-med to put under my tongue. This is to calm me. I am still nervous. I am hoping and praying that all goes well. A million things are running through my mind and my emotions are high. A few hours later, Daine is almost finished giving his second bag of stem cells and the nurse comes in to give me a sedative injection. The doctor walks in and behind her are the two bags. I find it strange that the bone-marrow transplant is a drip procedure.

The first bag is attached to my J-line. 'Now all we do is wait', says Dr. Nel. Mom comes and sits with me. I can vaguely hear what she is saying. My body starts to feel all tingly. No pain, just discomfort. I fall into a light sleep but am still fully aware of my surroundings. I wake up and Dr. Nel is putting up the next bag. The first drop enters where the last drop ended. I am beginning to develop a slight headache but it's nothing serious. I feel strange. A few hours later the last drop enters my body. I am told to rest for the remainder of the evening. I fall asleep peacefully with mom by my side.

The next morning I wake up and realise it's over. I am ecstatic but too tired to jump up and scream. Everyone comes in to say congratulations. I'm still not completely out of danger. The next few days are critical and I will have to be closely monitored. Mom is on the phone with dad and everyone. It's such a happy time. I wish I could just run out into the streets and celebrate. The doctors are relieved and I feel overwhelmed. A few days later dad comes up to see us and to fetch Daine. The transplant is a huge success. My body starts to get stronger every day. I long for the day that I can leave the isolation ward. We are all so much happier. Mom and I have lots to talk about now. Our journey has taken a whole year and we are so grateful to have come to this point. All those painful months and we are finally seeing the light.

Chapter 9

Recuperation period

THE transplant is over and now my body has to recuperate. I know it's not over yet but at least we can be positive and know that we are almost there. I'm finally taken out of isolation. This is one of the happiest moments of my life. I'm finished with chemo, had the transplant and now I'm released from isolation. I have mom by my side as I'm put in a wheel chair. They put a mask over my nose and mouth in order to block out as many germs as possible as I go from a sterile area to a general ward. I smile at the nurses as the porter wheels me away. I can see they feel my joy. I am just so happy to be out of isolation that I don't really care where I am. I am now referred to a different doctor. Every day I still receive medication and my appetite is improving. Mom notices that I have developed a bit of a cough but I think nothing of it. I'm craving a pie and mom goes to the shop downstairs and buys food for us. I start to feel like my old self again. Then night falls and the body pains begin again. I've been taken off the morphine and pethadene and can feel the pain they were disguising. The nurses are only allowed to give me Panado. I cry myself to sleep for a few nights.

Mom has to go home for a while. I am out of the critical stage and I feel strong, so she leaves. I have made friends with the lady who lies opposite me in the ward. She has cancer in her throat. It's very sad. We walk to the shop together as I grow stronger by the day. As I walk along the passages, holding the walls to balance, we pass many people who all stare at us. The shop is situated near the entrance to the hospital, so all the people walking in and out catch our eye. I feel like a freak. I feel angry. We walk back and sit in our beds chatting again. The ward has a beautiful view. I would look out of the window at the trees. I miss everyone dearly. I cry and cry, longing for the day that mom would say she was on her way back. I just want to go home. They phone every day but that isn't enough for me.

The reason I am still in hospital is because I have had some complications after the transplant. I developed a lung infection that causes me to cough all the time and feel ill again. This goes on for weeks. I wake up one morning feeling strange. I'm not hungry but I want to eat. I'm hungry in my mind and my stomach is growling but I can't swallow anything. I call mom from the phone box and ask her to please come back. She says they're on their way and will be with me in the morning. A girl offers me a banana, I try to eat it but it won't go down. I inform the doctors and they say it's normal for me to lose my appetite after this whole traumatic experience. I then had to get a pipe up my nose and into my stomach to be able to get nutrients into my body. It was terrible. Mom and dad finally come up and I am so happy to see them that I start to cry. Mom immediately notices that I've changed and I bring them up to speed about my appetite.

I'm eventually let out of hospital to stay at the Kerkhuis. I have to come in for regular tests as an outpatient and also have to have an immune booster drip every week for three months. This means we are unable to go home and we have to stay in Cape Town in the Kerkhuis. I finally get to meet all the people in the house and it's nice to be able to walk around and not be in hospital. Dad, mom and I decide to go to the Spur to celebrate me being out of hospital. We decide to walk as it isn't far from the Kerkhuis but for me it feels like we have been walking for hours. I order a hamburger. The owner comes over to speak to us and she says I can have anything I want on the menu for free. I prefer the simpler things now, so I stick to a hamburger. When it arrives it looks so yummy but my appetite is still gone. I force a bit down but I'm really not ready to eat. Dad could only stay for a while and had to return home again.

The next three months seem so long. The Kerkhuis becomes our new home and we spend many days and nights chatting to our house-mates and the owner. We meet many interesting people who also have problems and are staying there because a loved one is in at Groote Schuur hospital. It is a blessing to be able to talk to these people and maybe even help them with some words of encouragement. Our room is upstairs and dad often comes to visit with the boys. We walk to the Spar and to the mall, trying our best to be a normal family again. It's tough to walk and I have to hold onto them.

Mom and I were getting fed up with not being able to go home. Mom and I continue to go to the hospital every week. We have to see Professor Norvinski. He is the head of the Hematology and Oncology department. He speaks to us about my future treatment. I will have to be on contraceptives for the rest of my life as I could get Osteoporosis due to my weakened bones. I'm not allowed to be in crowded places for the next couple of months and should avoid being in the presence of smokers. This is a difficult rule as both my parents smoke. He also said that I should be careful not to get too emotionally upset as it can trigger one of the bad cells again. We go downstairs to get my immune booster, which is given via a drip. It is a bottle of yellowish liquid, which is attached to my J-line. The doctors and nurses are really friendly and sweet. The nurses are always chatting about their weekends and it makes us laugh every time.

The three months drag on until finally it's time to remove my J-line as my immune boosters are complete. This operation will take place in Port Elizabeth so we are free to go home. *Wow!* We are so excited. We get home and dad fetches us from the airport. I will have to go back to get bone-marrow biopsy's once a month, then every three months, six months and eventually only once a year. It's great to be home and I spend as much time with my family as possible. It took me over nine months to recuperate properly as I was very weak.

I had to do something about my education. We went to my old school to ask if I could do Grade 11 & 12 in one year. I was afraid that I would be too old in matric if I did it over two years. They declined our request and so I went to apply at Damelin Correspondence. I did that for four months but unfortunately it became too difficult for me to study without a teacher. I had been out of school for so long.

When I finally got home everyone's life had continued as normal without me. I had missed out on so much. I turned nineteen that year. My level of maturity superseded that of my peers. I had a different view of life compared to them. I went out a few times with my cousins and mingled with my old friends. One even came up to me and said 'I thought you were dead.' It was a huge shock to hear that coming from someone I knew. It made me realise who my real friends were.

I eventually went on to study hair dressing. I worked in my aunt's salon full-time and studied part-time, every Tuesday. The course was a bit boring and was for a three year period. I could not see myself moving so slowly, and I did not even know what I really wanted out of life. I always wanted to do something great, something special and creative. Maybe one day it will come to me.

I have always been interested in modeling and have done a few shoots here and there but I never 'made it big.' I started my own model agency in Port Elizabeth called Blaze Models and I hope that it will prosper. I want to help the Cancer Association through my company's achievements. I take life one day at a time. I try to laugh as much as possible, even though I do have moments of depression. One of my dream jobs would be to work as an air hostess and travel the world. I will never give up on my dreams. I will find myself someday.

A lot has changed since going through my ordeal, emotionally, mentally and physically. I have changed. During my time in hospital I had some supernatural experiences. Mom and dad went to Word of Faith Christian Centre and spoke to one of the deacons there. He called me that night and prayed for me over the phone. He spoke in tongues and then ended by telling me that God was already busy healing me, I would be healed in a year. On another occasion, in the early stage of my Groote Schuur hospital stay, a lady walked into my room while mom was not there. This did not surprise me as I would often receive gifts and visitors that knew of my story. She was a beautiful coloured lady. The only difference was that she walked in crying. She tried to speak but it seemed as though she could not hold back her tears. She took my hand and told me that she didn't know why she was there. I looked at her with curiosity.

She said 'I was sitting in my kitchen this morning and God spoke to me.' 'He told me that I should come and tell you not to be afraid anymore. He was healing you. One year.'

She gave me a hug and left. When mom returned I told her about the women. Nobody else saw her. That is something I will never be able to explain but I know in my heart who that women was. She was an angel, sent to me by God to give me an important message. A message that would give me hope. This happened the day after I had contemplated jumping out of the window. I was so sick of being sick. My hope was fading and God sent her to help me. The whole time I was there, I felt His presence. I knew He was right there guiding me through everything. Sometimes he held Shirley's hand and brought her to see us. Mom will tell you the same thing. I made a promise to God that if he saved me, I would spread his message and tell everyone in an attempt to save their lives as well. So here it is My Lord. I want to do everything in my power to spread the story of my miracle.

I travel up and down to Cape Town for bone-marrow biopsies and each time I am improving. On one of these trips mom and I travel up on the Greyhound bus. We arrive at the *Kerkhuis*, where we always stay. Everyone is happy to see us. The next day we go to the hospital. Dr. Littleton is so pleased to see how healthy I look. I have even put on weight.

He tells me about a boy who had just been diagnosed. His name is Shaun. Dr. Littleton asks if I could go and see him and talk to him about my procedure. I walk up to the wards with mom. It's difficult for us because we never wanted to go up there again. I put on the protective gear and wash my hands twice.

The tables are turned and I'm now the visitor. The difference is that I truly understand what Shaun is going through. He has been diagnosed with Leukemia and Lymphoma. His hair was shaved yet he looks pretty healthy to me. We chat for a while and he asks me a lot of questions. It's nice to know most of the answers.

Shaun and I became friends and I kept in contact with him as much as I could. I know, from my experience that sometimes you just want to be alone. Throughout my recuperation Shaun was going through his chemo. Eventually, he is released from hospital for a month before his transplant. Shaun's 12 year old brother is his bone-marrow match. One evening Daine and I went to talk to Shaun and his family about the transplant and what to expect. Daine chats to Shaun's brother about what he will have to go through. Shaun is looking so much better and his mom has a relieved look on her face. After his transplant he begins to look better and better and we keep in touch. His girlfriend is a sweet girl named Christine. She really loved him because she was there for him all the way and supported him. His hair grew back and he was doing so well.

One day I got a call that he was back in hospital. Shaun had relapsed. The cancer had come back. By this time Drs. Littleton and Nel had moved to Port Elizabeth and were working at the Provincial Hospital Hematology department. Shaun and his mom battled on for a few months until Shaun's fragile body couldn't take it anymore. I remember going for a checkup and as I walked out Shaun and his mom were getting out of the car. I gave him a big hug but I didn't know what to say. He was so positive. He had no fear in his eyes. He was just content.

A few days later Shaun Van Schalkwyk passed away. The funeral theme was pink. Dad went with me. It was the saddest day I had ever experienced. Everyone was crying. I know that Shaun is in Heaven and his story will be remembered forever. At 21 years old, this soldier went home. To his mom, I hope that you find peace. You are such a brave lady. Shaun will always be with you.

After Shaun died I realised that I had to help people. I had to spread my story. More and more young people, children and teenagers are being diagnosed with this disease and a number of them are from the Eastern Cape. It's important to listen to someone who doesn't feel well. Don't leave it until tomorrow. Go and have that 'full blood count.' It can be caught in time. To Eugene, Sanshcia, Darren, all friends of mine who have been diagnosed with leukemia or cancer. You guys know what it's about. You are all fighters from the Eastern Cape. We all had different experiences with a similar disease. All of us shared the same doctor, Dr. Neil Littleton, including Shaun.

I have been in remission since 2004 and I am still going strong. I do talks for the South African National Blood Service to keep blood donors motivated. It's so important that we help each other. If I can change one person's mind about donating blood, then I know I've done my job properly. The emotional reward I get from talking to people and telling my story is priceless. To the reader I hope that you found peace in reading this book. Smile a lot, love a lot and live, live as much as you can.

Choose to fight. Don't take anyone for granted. Life could change dramatically for you, so make sure you have no regrets. I know I don't.

Prayer

When loved ones walk into the sunset

And wave a last goodbye,

And sorrow's shadows deepen

And each smile becomes a sigh,

What a comfort and a solace

God's blessed words afford-

Though now absent from the body,

They will know no disappointment

When life's trials at last are done

Eternal bliss and joy await them

Just beyond the setting sun.

The bone-marrow donor
A letter in my brother's words at the age of 10 years old

To save my sister's life

When I heard the doctor say that my sister had AML Leukemia, I had no idea what that was or how serious it was. Straight away I heard my mom shout, 'Oh no that can't be' and then I looked at my dad and he had tears running down his face. I knew then that there was something terribly wrong with my sister and I began to cry. I saw my sister leave the room and I immediately followed her. I was so scared and didn't know what was going on.

I asked her, 'Chanel, are you going to die?' she looked at me and replied, 'I don't know.' I burst into tears right there as I didn't want my sister to die.

My sister had to leave for Cape Town as soon as possible, along with my mom. I went home with my dad and asked him all sorts of questions. I also asked my dad if Chanel would die and he said 'No boy just keep praying for your sister.' I continued going to school but my heart was so sore and I was frightened as I didn't know if I would see my sister again. I attended Parsons Hill Primary School at the time. My Principal Mr. Sadler was such a great and kind man as were the teachers.

My father had explained to my brother and me that Chanel needed to have a bone marrow transplant and that we both needed to be tested. We didn't know straight away if either one of us was a match but once again dad told us to pray. I went to school the following day and when school came out my dad was waiting to meet me. I was surprised as I normally walked home. Dad gave me a big smile and said, 'climb in, boy, I have very good news for you.' He told me that I was a match for my sister and that I would be going to Cape Town at the end of the week. I was so very happy because I knew that I would be able to save my sister. My principal and teachers were so kind; they collected money for us and also packed us a lot of sweets for the bus ride. When I walked into the hospital I had a funny feeling in my stomach, I was excited that I would see my sister again but also so scared as I didn't know what to expect. I wanted to give her a big hug and she started to cry when she saw me.

Chanel asked me if I was scared to do this and I said no but deep down inside I was terrified. I didn't want her to worry about me. My dad went back home as he had to get back to work. I went to stay with my mom at the Kerkhuis. The doctor gave my mom injection needles with special stuff that she had to inject me with to build up my cells. This had to happen for one week. I was so tired when my mom would wake me up and say, 'come boy it's time for another injection.' My mom used to cry so much at the time as it was so sore for me, it used to burn like hell. I hated it but every time I new it was to save my sister's life. The doctors then tested me to see if my cells had grown and they were happy as it was a great success.

I was given a small pill that would make me a bit drowsy. Dad, mom and I went to the cafeteria to get something to eat. I started to feel all funny and called to my dad and told him I couldn't feel my legs. I don't remember much after that, except that they placed a long screw in my spine. I screamed and screamed.

I had to have a catheter in my upper leg that burned so much once it was in. My mom just kept crying, I used to wonder if my mom's tears would dry up as all she did was cry. When I asked if she was okay she would smile and say, 'yes boy I am fine. I am just so proud of you.'

All I want to say is that I pray every night and thank the Lord for giving my sister back to us. If this ever happens to you, just remember that God is with you and always pray, have faith. I have learnt a great lesson from this terrible experience and that is to appreciate one another as you never realise what you have until it's gone.

Say I love you every day.

God Bless,

Daine Wewege

A letter from my Mother

*T*HE *pain, the sadness, every breath taken with hope, prayer and faith and yet so frightened. These were the mixed feelings going on inside of my beautiful daughter, feelings that I wanted to wipe out. I wanted to assure my child that there was no need for these scary seconds that had come and gone, yet it seemed that moment would never come. It all started with a 'big bang' in our hearts. This I would never have expected.*

Let me start at the beginning. My own mother had always come to visit me on a Saturday. She was my best friend, and my anchor in life. She had been complaining that she had not been feeling well. I had suggested that she get some vitamins. My sister-in-law decided to take her to see a doctor. That day my wonderful mother was diagnosed with lung cancer. I had come home from work and was busy preparing supper for my family when my brother, sister-in-law and mother arrived.

My mother wanted to see me alone in the bedroom. When she told me the news, I thought I had gone paralysed. I was numb but remember screaming, 'no, no! This cannot be true.' My strong wonderful mother said that I must not be so upset, that she would still live for a long time and would be here with me. Here was my mother, just diagnosed with cancer and yet she was trying to be strong for me and comforting me. That was the way she was. I explained to my children what was wrong with their grandmother and they had also shed tears of sadness, they loved her so much. Chanel took the news very badly.

Chanel was diagnosed with AML Leukemia about a month after my mother's diagnosis When the doctor broke the news to my husband and me, I thought I was going to die. I could not have another loved one taken from me. My husband Johnny was in shock and tears just rolled down his face. He held his little girl and cried with her and said, 'don't be scared, you will be okay. You're daddy's little girl. We love you so much and we are all here for you. Daddy doesn't have money but even if we have to get the best doctors for you, that's what we'll do.'

We didn't realise it then but we already had the best doctors. Chanel had been booked into St. George's straight away as there was no time to waste. My beautiful child was so pale, so afraid and so weak. All I wanted to do was hold her and take it all away but I couldn't. I had no control over this disease I felt so much hurt in my heart.

The following day we took my mother to see the doctor at the Provincial Hospital to find out how far the cancer was and if she could get treatment. We waited in the corridor. I still remember a cold wind blowing through the passage where we sat. My mother took my hand and squeezed it, giving me a smile of reassurance. The doctor called us in and Mom sat on the bed and I put my arms around her. The doctor told her that she did not have long to live and that the cancer had spread and there was no possibility of her having treatment. I felt blind as the tears blocked my sight but when I blinked and looked at my mom, she smiled and said 'thank you, doctor, I just want to know: will I make Christmas with my children?'

He replied 'enjoy every moment with your family now'. As we got outside there was a light drizzle falling and my mom put her arms around me and sang, 'rain drops are falling on my head' and she laughed and gave me a hug. How could someone who had just been told that her time was nearly up, sing and laugh? This was all for me, I know she was frightened inside but would not break down in front of me.

My mother went to live with my brother and sister-in-law as I had to leave with my child for Cape Town, Tygerburg Hospital. I went to say goodbye to my mom and told her that I would be back soon to take care of her. All she kept saying was look after my child (Chanel), take care of that girl and be strong for her, she will make it. She thought of Chanel as her own daughter and loved her so much. I never saw my mother again. She died soon after that. I had gone down to Port Elizabeth to bury her, but had to rush back as Chanel was so ill and in so much pain. From then on, I was a walking dummy. I was hurt, confused and so worried about my child. I knew I had to be strong, she needed me and I also knew there would come a time for me to mourn but right now I had to be there for my beautiful daughter.

Seeing my child in so much pain, so sad and so weak was terribly hard. I couldn't show her how scared and how worried I was. I often asked myself 'will my child walk out here with me one day, or will I walk out alone?' I slept, ate and lived with this question every second of every day. No one can really understand what it's like to see your daughter fading away in front of you unless you go through it yourself. There came a time when Chanel had to have an oxygen mask on 24 hours a day. I would sit there watching her gasping for air through the mask. I was dying every day, bit by bit seeing what she had to go through and there was nothing I could do but pray. We prayed so much together, she was so weak but always told me 'mom don't worry, God won't dish out something that you can't handle. God's got his angels looking after me.' Here was my child, so weak, so sick yet trying to reassure me that all would be well. Time was going on and all we had was hope, faith and our love for each other. I believe that the love we carry in our hearts is also there to heal each other's pain. I missed my husband and other children, my two sons.

Sheldon was 16 and the baby, Daine was nine years old. I would call them and they would ask when would it be time for Chanel and me to come home. Daine was the match as a marrow donor for Chanel. 'Thank you Lord for yet another blessing.' I will never forget what my thin, tiny little boy, looked like while lying in the hospital bed with pipes coming out of his groin while his marrow was collected for his sister, who was lying upstairs. He lay downstairs and Chanel was upstairs on the fourth floor. I was sitting next to my boy, holding his hand and telling him how sorry mommy was that he had to go through all this pain. The answer I got from a nine year old child was 'mommy, I will do this again if I can save my sister's life.'

I burst into tears and gave this little angel a hug. I then ran upstairs to watch the marrow going into Chanel. I held her hand and said, 'be strong my sweetheart the long sad, dark days are nearly over,' but all she wanted to know how Daine was. I told her to be positive as her little brother had just told me that he would do it again to save her life. My beautiful daughter smiled at me with tears running down her cheeks. She was so beautiful even though she was so thin and her cheek bones stuck out.

She is my angel and I believe God has given her back to me and all of us in order for her to be there for others. Never hold back when you can reach out and help, love and pray for others. There were many times I was angry with God and asked Him 'what are you doing? Why are you doing this to me? You have taken my mommy away from me and now you want to take my daughter? Why?'

Today I understand and I asked God for forgiveness for doubting him, as I did so many times during those terrible agonising months. I believe that He let my mom and Chanel get sick together. He knew when my mother passed away I would have gone off my head. I would never ever have handled it but with Chanel ill at the time, I had to be strong for her. If I were to give up then my child would also have given up. God has a reason for everything, we don't see it straight away but after a while we realise God is only looking out for us as He loves us all so much.

I would like to say a few words to the families out there that have a loved one suffering from any illness. Have faith, pray and most of all be there for each other no matter how bad things get. Remember love is a gift we have received from God. The Lord has blessed us so that we can love each other and never stop telling each other that, it costs nothing to say 'I love you.'

Shireen Wewege

A tribute to my Dad

Johnny Wewege: 1965 - 2012

THE morning of January 24th 2012 started out like any other. I got up, brushed my teeth and got ready for work. This morning would be a little bit different as I was scheduled to do make-up on the lovely Christina Storm for a music video. As soon as I got to work I called my mom to tell her how it went. Sitting at the reception of Maritime Motors I went about my normal routine, unaware of how my day would turn out.

At around 15:30 p.m. I received a frantic phone call from my mom. She told me that my dad had been involved in an accident at work. A batch of steel had fallen on top of him, from a dangerous height. Panic started to flow through my veins as I felt the pit of my stomach go hollow. I jumped from my desk and ran to my manager and told him I needed to leave immediately. They assisted me as best they could and before long I was driven to Greenacres Hospital by Neil, a dear friend and a driver at Maritime Motors. Throughout the drive he tried to calm me down. I couldn't stop crying and thinking the worst. I asked him to stop at my mom's house to pick up my little brother Daine, who was also frantic. We ran into the emergency room and mom rose up to greet us, tears streaming from her eyes.

'Where is dad?' I asked.

Two of his colleagues were there with the Injury on Duty (IOD) forms that needed to be handed in at reception. I wondered how long it had taken them to bring him here. There were conflicting reports to what had actually happened.

The nurse called my mom. She was finally able to speak to my dad. Evie, my dad's mom arrived and straight after her my Uncle Mark, Aunty Jean, Uncle Wayne, Aunty Therisa, all my dad's siblings along with the rest of their families. Mom came out while they wheeled dad off to get x-rays. Evie watched wasn't given the chance to talk to him. Mom came back to relay what he had said. He had grabbed her wrist and held her close, telling her he was not going to make it as he could feel his insides moving around.

We called Sheldon, who was working out of town. He came as soon as he could. Eventually the medical staff realised dad had internal bleeding and he had to go into surgery immediately. For four long hours we paced around, praying in a room together, hoping for a bit of grace. It was the worst night of my entire life. When the surgical doors opened and they wheeled him into intensive care I ran to the nurse who told me that the surgery had gone well. Without a second thought, I ran down stairs to tell Uncle Wayne, Sheldon and Daine and everyone else that he was going to be OK.

Celebrations erupted through the parking lot. We all took turns to walk in and see him in Intensive Care. A large steel apparatus held his insides together connecting his hip bones to his stomach. I gasped at the sight and the nurse covered him quickly. Everyone had a turn to see him, to speak to him and to hold his hand.

My beautiful dad, the pain he must have been going through, the thoughts that must have been running through his mind. After about two hours we thought he would make it through the night. We were talking about leaving and coming back in the morning when the nurse stopped us and told us it wouldn't be much longer. The pain of those words stabbed us all. Everyone ran into the ICU ward and started to pray frantically.

Sheldon vomited next to the bed as he screamed out, pleading for my dad not to *leave us*. Mom knelt down next to him talking to him like she always did, calling him 'my boy'. Evie was screaming out for the healing of God, as her son slipped further and further away. I put my hands on dad and shouted out in prayer through my tears. His blood pressure dropped to 40. Uncle Wayne was crying as well, his only brother, soon to be taken. Aunty Therisa ran home, unable to handle the pain. Daine, my 17 year old brother begged this not to be true.

I called for the nurses to do something but the doctors had already left. They gave him some more blood. His blood pressure rose and then fell again. Fifteen minutes later he was really gone. The blood pressure machine showed 0.

From what we can gather, he wasn't even on his side of the factory at Steel Pipes and Fittings in Port Elizabeth, that day. A steel band snapped causing a bunch of steel pipes to tumble on top of my father, crushing his pelvis in seven different places and severing the artery in his groin. There is never a reason for such a tragedy to occur and to this day we ask God why he took our dad, our son, our brother, our friend at the age of 46? He had already been through the tragedy of seeing his daughter almost die. I suppose we will never know the answer to that until the day we are also taken to Heaven to be with him again.

We love you, Daddy, and I think about you every single day. We miss you so much. Your memory will always live on. Till we meet again.

Thank you, from Chanel

THE bone-marrow fluid is a milky, light-brown substance. I find it hard to believe that it's derived naturally from the body of my nine year old brother. It took him nine years to create this life-saving potion that would one day save his sister's life. Only God could have created such craftsmanship, such an amazing machine that could make a person out of a single sperm and egg cell. A structure so magnificent that it can aid in saving another human being. One bag down and one to go. The doctor carefully attaches the next bag of stem cells to my J-line. It doesn't hurt; it's just uncomfortable as this foreign substance becomes part of me, as it flows through me, as it heals me. I become exhausted and start to fade away. I can hear voices speaking but I want to sleep. I am still in danger. At any time my body can reject this new bone-marrow, like an army defending its turf. The next day it almost feels as if I have been born again. My parents are ecstatic and the doctors gasp a sigh of relief. They have managed to save yet another life through the healing power of God and medical science. The modesty shown by these phenomenal human beings is breathtaking. I thank them for their knowledge and for fighting for me.

Thank you, Daine, my little brother, you mean the world to me. You are part of me now. My little bone-marrow donor! I thank my parents, Shireen (mom for carrying me through that hospital experience step-by-step) and sadly, in loving memory of John Wewege, daddy. I miss you each and every day. Please say 'hi' to Shirls for me. To my brother Sheldon thank you for your support and love and all the letters you wrote to me while you were at school and I was in hospital. God gave me a beautiful family and I know that this journey pulled us all closer together. To the rest of my supportive family, thank you. I hope you all know how special you are to me. It is impossible for me to name you all.

To my wonderful Doctors:
Dr. Gregory Musson (St George's Hospital, Port Elizabeth), You cared for me from the beginning of my journey.

Dr. Schmidt and Dr. Els (Tygerburg Hospital X-Block, Cape Town), for helping me through the tough days.

Dr. Neil Littleton and Dr. Nel (Grooteschuur Cape Town / Provincial hospital, Oncology, Port Elizabeth).

The isolation and transplant stages. To the doctors that have slipped my mind, you know who you are, thank you.

To Dr. Swart (Greenacres Hospital), who took the time to notice me on that first day when this all started. You are the reason I was saved in time.

To Dr. Wickens (Greenacres Hospital), who was my diagnostic doctor and dealt with me from the point of the discovery of my disease.

The subtle honesty and kindness of the nurses and their loving touch meant so much to me. You, ladies, were my precious little angels and I hope you know how important you all are.

To the SANBS crew for doing such a great job at raising awareness for blood donations. You are the *'lifeblood'* of the medical process that made my recovery possible.

Thank you, God. I know you have a plan for my life. I know this book is meant to be and it will help others get through their journey. Thank you for the courage you have given me to write these pages – the strength to reach for those painful memories and express them to the world.